ESTIMATING DRUG REQUIREMENTS: A PRACTICAL MANUAL

ACTION PROGRAMME ON ESSENTIAL DRUGS

WORLD HEALTH ORGANIZATION GENEVA

First Edition, 1988
Reprinted, 1990, 1991

CBS

CBS Publishers & Distributors Pvt. Ltd.

New Delhi • Bengaluru • Chennai • Kochi • Kolkata • Mumbai
Hyderabad • Nagpur • Patna • Pune • Vijayawada

ISBN: 81-239-0357-X

Authorised Reprint: 1993

Published by **Satish Kumar Jain** and produced by **Varun Jain** for
CBS Publishers & Distributors Pvt. Ltd.,
4819/XI Prahlad Street, 24 Ansari Road, Daryaganj, New Delhi - 110002
delhi@cbspd.com, cbspubs@airtelmail.in • www.cbspd.com
Ph.: 23289259, 23266861, 23266867 • Fax: 011-23243014

Corporate Office: 204 FIE, Industrial Area, Patparganj, Delhi - 110 092
Ph: 49344934 • Fax: 011-49344935
E-mail: publishing@cbspd.com • publicity@cbspd.com

Branches:
- ***Bengaluru:*** 2975, 17th Cross, K.R. Road, Bansankari 2nd Stage, Bengaluru - 70 • Ph: +91-80-26771678/79 • Fax: +91-80-26771680 E-mail: cbsbng@gmail.com, bangalore@cbspd.com
- ***Chennai:*** No. 7, Subbaraya Street, Shenoy Nagar, Chennai - 600030 Ph: +91-44-26681266, 26680620 • Fax: +91-44-42032115 E-mail: chennai@cbspd.com
- ***Kochi:*** Ashana House, 39/1904, A.M. Thomas Road, Valanjambalam, Ernakulum, Kochi • Ph: +91-484-4059061-65 Fax: +91-484-4059065 • E-mail: cochin@cbspd.com
- ***Kolkata:*** 6-B, Ground Floor, Rameshwar Shaw Road, Kolkata - 700014 Ph: +91-33-22891126/7/8 • E-mail: kolkata@cbspd.com
- ***Mumbai:*** 83-C, Dr. E. Moses Road, Worli, Mumbai - 400018 Ph: +91-9833017933, 022-24902340/41 • E-mail: mumbai@cbspd.com

Representatives:
- Hyderabad: 0-9885175004
- Patna: 0-9334159340
- Jharkhand: 0-9811541605
- Nagpur: 0-9021734563
- Pune: 0-9623451994
- Uttarakhand: 0-9716462459

Printed at:
J.S. Offset Printers, Delhi (India)

PREFACE

This manual was written by Mr Adrian Griffiths, Director of Research of the Health Management Institute (HMI), Geneva, under a contractual service agreement between HMI and the World Health Organization Action Programme on Essential Drugs and Vaccines (DAP).

The content of the manual was developed by an informal working group which met five times during 1984-1987, and in work done between meetings, including field tests in several countries. The members of the working group were:

Consultants

Mr Adrian Griffiths, Director of Research, Health Management Institute, Geneva.
Dr Hans Hogerzeil, Associate Professional Officer, World Health Organization, Eastern Mediterranean Regional Office.*
Dr Jonathan Quick, Director of Drug Management Programmes, Management Sciences for Health, Boston, USA.
Dr Godfrey Walker, Senior Lecturer, London School of Hygiene and Tropical Medicine, U.K. **
Dr James Wolff, Project Officer, Management Sciences for Health, Boston, USA.

WHO Secretariat

Mrs Margaretha Helling-Borda, Senior Scientist, Action Programme on Essential Drugs and Vaccines, WHO, Geneva.
Mrs Ramona Lunt, Scientist, Action Programme on Essential Drugs and Vaccines, WHO, Geneva.
Mr Ed Dowd, Chief, Epidemiological and Statistical Methodology, WHO, Geneva.***

The valuable advice of staff working in relevant technical programmes of WHO has been incorporated into Module 5 which includes illustrative standard drug treatment schedules for quantification of drug requirements based on average doses.

The preparation of the manual was financed by grants from the Directorate of Development Cooperation and Humanitarian Aid, Switzerland, the Swedish International Development Authority/Swedish Agency for Research Cooperation with Developing Countries (SIDA/SAREC), and from Interpharma, the association of the Swiss pharmaceutical companies Ciba-Geigy, Hoffmann-La Roche, and Sandoz.

* Now Technical Officer, Action Programme on Essential Drugs and Vaccines, WHO, Geneva.
** Now Manager, Safe Motherhood Research Programme, WHO, Geneva.
*** Now retired.

TABLE OF CONTENTS

LIST OF TABLES

LIST OF TABLES
(Continued)

PART I

INTRODUCTION

MODULE 1:
OBJECTIVES AND USE OF THE MANUAL

1. INTRODUCTION

Effective health care requires a judicious balance of preventive and curative services. This manual deals with a crucial and often deficient input to curative services: an adequate supply of appropriate drugs.

The manual is intended primarily for countries embarking on an Action Programme on Essential Drugs and Vaccines, which requires an effective drug supply management system. The main components of such a system are:

(1)	**SELECTION**	deciding what drugs are needed.
(2)	**QUANTIFICATION**	estimating how much of each drug is needed.
(3)	**PROCUREMENT**	selecting suppliers, placing and monitoring orders, checking delivery quantities and quality, and paying suppliers.
(4)	**DISTRIBUTION**	reception, storage, stock control, transportation, and record keeping for monitoring and control.
(5)	**USE**	prescription, dispensing and use of drugs, and patients' compliance with prescriptions.

This manual deals with the second component, quantification. **Quantification should not be regarded as a purely computational procedure**, for as can be seen above, it is part of a sequence of interdependent steps in the drug supply management system. Effective quantification requires specific data concerning morbidity and drug use, and fundamental decisions about which drugs are to be available and how they are to be prescribed. In short, the process must be fully integrated into the drug supply management system. This integration can only be assured if there is **a long term and high level commitment** to an overall system based on an agreed policy and specific procedures.

In most countries, the quantification of drug requirements is based on past experience, short term reactions to crises, and subjective impressions of the quantities needed. In principle, such an approach can lead to progressive adjustment and refinement over the years, until the supply matches the demands of the health services, and these in turn match the morbidity of the population they serve.

In practice, the lack of systematic procedures based on morbidity and the use of health services, the absence of a clinical and economic consensus about the most cost-effective treatments, and pressures from various sources have made such progressive improvement difficult. Inadequate quantification is a particularly serious problem in developing countries. Budgets are generally severely limited while many countries are highly dependent on imports; orders have to be placed well in advance and paid for in scarce foreign exchange. Mistakes are difficult and expensive to correct, and can seriously reduce the effectiveness of the health services.

2. THE TWO METHODS OF QUANTIFICATION

This manual presents two methods for quantifying drug requirements. For both methods examples of calculations are given using short essential drug lists for the middle level (health centre) and the first (community health worker) level of health care. The two methods presented are:

(1) **THE PATIENT MORBIDITY-STANDARD TREATMENT METHOD,** called the morbidity method for short from here on.

(2) **THE ADJUSTED CONSUMPTION METHOD**, called the consumption method for short from here on.

Both methods are based on data concerning the actual (or projected) use of health services. Their purpose is **to ensure that the health services concerned have adequate drug supplies to treat their case load of patients.**

The quantities estimated by these two methods are less than would be needed to treat all the morbidity in the population. Such quantities could in theory be calculated from population based morbidity data, but this basis of calculation is not used in the manual for three reasons:

(a) the necessary population morbidity data are rarely available, and are difficult or costly to collect;

(b) not all morbidity results in a demand for health services;

(c) the extent to which demands can be met is itself limited by the availability of health services.

The basic principles of the two methods are summarized below. Both methods require that:

(a) **the drugs to be included should already have been selected for each type of facility whose requirements are being estimated, and**

(b) **there is a basic consensus about the appropriate use of these drugs.** As will be explained later, for the morbidity method this consensus is explicitly formulated in standard treatment protocols.

2.1 The patient morbidity-standard treatment method

This method starts from two sets of data:

(a) **the number of episodes of each health problem** treated by the type or types of facilities for which drug requirements are to be estimated;

(b) **average standard treatment schedules** agreed for each health problem defined.

The quantity of drugs given as a standard treatment for each health problem, multiplied by the number of treatment episodes of that problem, gives the total quantity of drugs required for it.

Quantity of the drug specified for a standard course of treatment	x	Number of treatment episodes of the health problem	=	Total quantity of a drug required for a given health problem

This calculation is repeated for each health problem and its corresponding drugs. Where a drug is used for more than one health problem, the respective totals are added together to obtain the total quantity required. These quantities may then be divided by the total number of treatment episodes of all kinds, expressed in thousands, to give the average drug requirements per 1,000 treatment episodes. Different versions of this method have been used in several countries in recent years (2-5,8).

2.2 The adjusted consumption method

This method starts from existing consumption of the drugs concerned. For each type of health facility, a number of "standard" facilities are identified, which have a reasonably representative workload, acceptable drug supply, and rational prescribing and consumption. Their drug consumption is reviewed, and for any drug whose consumption is considered inappropriate, the quantity is adjusted upwards or downwards to an appropriate level. The adjusted quantities of drugs used per "standard" facility are converted into standard quantities per 1000 treatment episodes, and these are then used to estimate the drug quantities required for each facility of the type concerned, according to its expected number of treatment episodes, as in the previous method. One of the most comprehensive applications of this method to date is the quantification procedure developed for mission hospitals and health centres in Ghana (6, 7).

3. TARGET GROUP OF THE MANUAL

This manual is intended for **staff responsible for the quantification of drug requirements at national or regional level.** In practice this usually means a multidisciplinary team of pharmacists, physicians, administrators and epidemiologists, familiar with drug management procedures and the use of epidemiological data.

4. OBJECTIVES OF THE MANUAL

The ultimate objectives of quantifying drug requirements are to ensure that appropriate drugs are available to treat the expected case load at each health facility and, more broadly, to promote and maintain the rational and economic use of drugs.

Specific objectives

The objective of this manual is to develop practical competence in estimating the quantities of essential drugs needed at national or regional level, by type of health facility, using the two methods outlined above. Specifically, the manual aims to develop practical competence to:

(1) Assess the **need** for more systematic quantification of drug requirements.

(2) Set specific **practical objectives** for estimating drug requirements.

(3) Choose the most appropriate **method(s)** to use.

(4) Decide **what health problems are to be treated** at different types of facility.

(5) Prepare or review **essential drug lists.**

(6) Prepare or review **standard drug treatment schedules** for quantifying drug requirements, based on average doses (morbidity method only).

(7) Collect appropriate **morbidity and drug use data** from routine sources, or where necessary through special estimates.

(8) Calculate future **drug quantities** required.

(9) Calculate the **cost** of the estimated drug quantities.

(10) Plan **budget allocations** and **reconcile** estimated quantities to fit within the available budget.

(11) Use the final estimates to **order drugs** from suppliers and to issue them to health facilities.

(12) Evaluate the **effectiveness** of the quantification.

(13) **Refine estimates** in successive periods.

(14) Incorporate the quantification procedure into the **routine** management procedures of the drug supply system.

These objectives also imply improving awareness of:

(a) the costs and effects of existing prescribing habits;

(b) the importance of choosing and using the most rational and cost effective treatments;

(c) the importance of collecting appropriate and accurate routine data on patient morbidity and drug use.

5. USING THE MANUAL

The manual is in three parts. **Part I** contains an introduction to quantification, and the overall plan of work for quantifying drug requirements. **Part II** explains the patient morbidity-standard treatment method of quantification, and **Part III** explains the adjusted consumption method. Each method is divided into modules dealing in sequence with the individual steps involved. Each step is first explained, then illustrated by a practical example, including important components such as the health problem listing (Module 4) and the average standard treatment schedules (Module 5), and followed by a practical exercise as a self check on your understanding.

5.1 Use for self tuition

If you intend to use the manual for self tuition, the best approach is simply to work through it systematically doing the exercises which accompany each step. **Do not try to work too fast.**

In addition to the introduction, Part I also explains certain key decisions, which are required before quantification can begin, but are not part of the quantification process itself. (Decisions on what types of health problems are to be treated at each type of facility or level of care, and on their essential drug lists.) These inputs are very important and must be clearly understood before starting the actual quantification process, so all readers should read Part I. The exercises in Part I are optional, and no answers are given or can be given, for they vary according to the circumstances of each country. You will nevertheless find them a useful preparation for Parts II and III.
The exercises in Part II and III should be worked through in detail, so that you can check whether you have understood the calculation procedure before going on to the next Module. The arithmetic has been kept to a minimum and answers are given to each exercise.

5.2 Use for courses

The manual may also be used as the basis of a training course on the quantification of drug requirements. In principle, such a course should not require more than three days. An indicative schedule is given below:

	DAY 1:
9:00	Opening and introduction of participants.Introduction of the manual and the objectives of the course (Module l).
10:00	Assessing the need for quantification (Module 2).
11:00	Break.
11:30	Preparing an action plan (Module 3).
12:30	Lunch.
2:00	Preparing an action plan - continued (exercises).
4:00	End of day 1. (Hand out modules 5 and 6 to be read in preparation for day 2).
	DAY 2:
9:00	Listing and allocation of health problems by level of care, and selection of essential drug lists (Module 4).
10:30	Break.
11:00	Introduction to the morbidity method and average standard drug treatment schedules for quantification of drug requirements (Modules 4 and 5).
12:30	Lunch.
2:00	Average standard drug treatment schedules - continued.
3:30	Break.
4:00	Patient morbidity statistics and data collection Module 6).
5:30	End of day 2. (Hand out Modules 7 and 8 to be read in preparation for day 3).
	DAY 3:
9:00	The morbidity method (Module 7).
11:00	Break.
11:30	The morbidity method - continued.
12:30	Lunch.
2:00	The consumption method (Module 8).
3:30	Break.
4:00	The consumption method - continued.
5:00	End of course.

The quantification and costing calculations can be done on a micro-computer using a spreadsheet programme.

If computer based calculations are to be taught during the course, they can be used within the framework outlined above if course members are familiar with the use of computers and spreadsheets. Otherwise, it is advisable to have a fourth day devoted to the use of the computer for the calculations, so that the method is first clearly understood before embarking on the separate task of learning how to use a computer spreadsheet.

REFERENCES

(1) Management Sciences for Health, Managing drug supply, The selection, procurement, distribution, and use of pharmaceuticals in primary health care. Boston, Management Sciences for Health, 1982.

(2) Simmonds SP and Walker GJA. Essential drugs for primary health care standard packages. Lancet 1982; 1:435-6.

(3) WHO, WHO Emergency Health Kit. Standard drugs and clinic equipment for 10,000 persons for 3 months. Geneva, World Health Organization, 1983.

(4) Moore GD, Essential drugs for Kenya's rural population. World Health Forum 1982; 3:196-9.

(5) WHO, How to estimate essential drug requirements for the first time. Logistics and cold chain series, Geneva, World Health Organization.

(6) Hogerzeil HV, The use of essential drugs in Ghana. Int. J. Hlth. Serv. 1986; 16:425-40.

(7) Hogerzeil HV, Estimating drug requirements. Trop. Doct. 1986; 16:155-9.

(8) Helling-Borda M, Hogerzeil HV. Essential drugs for Democratic Yemen: estimating drug requirements. Alexandria, World Health Organization, 1986.

MODULE 2:

ASSESSING THE NEED FOR BETTER QUANTIFICATION

1. SYMPTOMS OF POOR QUANTIFICATION

As noted in Module 1, few countries have systematic procedures for quantifying drug requirements. This lack is particularly serious in developing countries because of their heavy dependence on imports, the need to plan orders well in advance, and the vital importance of making the best use of limited budgets and scarce foreign exchange.

The most commonly encountered symptoms of poor quantification of drug requirements are briefly described below. Of course these symptoms may be caused by several other deficiencies, but poor quantification is usually one of them and often the most important one.

1.1 Chronic and widespread shortages of commonly used drugs, despite adequate funding, procurement, and distribution.

1.2 Surpluses of a significant number of commonly used drugs or large surpluses of a smaller number of drugs usually mean that quantities have been overestimated. Sometimes overestimates are compounded by poor selection; the drugs involved are not appropriate to the morbidity pattern of the population, or are not in the form or dosage preferred by prescribers or by patients, and therefore remain unused.

For example, in a quantification exercise undertaken in Ghana, central decision makers considered quite rightly that a certain proportion of patients could just as well be treated with simpler, cheaper antibiotics as with more sophisticated and expensive ones. However, because prescribers were not at first involved in this decision, they continued to prescribe as before, and the reduced supplies of the sophisticated drugs ran out while the extra supplies of the simpler ones remained unused.

1.3 **Inequity of supply** between different levels of health services is also common; hospitals and urban based facilities are generally better supplied than rural based facilities. In extreme cases certain levels of service have regular surpluses whereas others have chronic shortages. Such inequities reflect factors like the greater influence of hospitals and the easier accessibility of urban facilities for delivering drugs, but they also often reflect a lack of proper quantification of the drugs required.

When such inequities arise, patients generally by-pass the appropriate but ill-supplied primary health care level, and go directly to higher level facilities, where they know drugs are available. These facilities are then overwhelmed with inappropriate cases and are unable to care for their intended case load as they should.

1.4 **Inadequate cost-effectiveness** by failure to use cheaper but equally effective drugs or dosage forms is a widespread problem. For example, expensive broad spectrum antibiotics are used when much cheaper penicillin would be just as effective for most patients, the more expensive broad spectrum drugs being reserved for resistant cases. Similarly, injectables and other expensive forms are often used where cheaper tablet forms would suffice.

1.5 **Irrational adjustments to budgetary constraints** may lead to irrational order quantities. If the reduction of order quantities to fit within budget is left to administrators unfamiliar with medical priorities, cuts tend to be made arbitrarily across the board, with little or no regard for priorities.

For example, if the budget is sufficient for only half the estimated requirements, a quite common reaction is simply to halve all order quantities. Such an adjustment would be logical only if all drugs were of equal importance, which of course is not the case. A cost-effectiveness oriented approach would cut less essential drugs first and most, and cut the more essential drugs least and only as a last resort.

1.6 **Irrational and ineffective prescribing** may also be caused by poor quantification of drug requirements. Prescribers faced with inadequate or inappropriate drug supplies usually either shorten treatments in an attempt to stretch their insufficient drug supplies as far as possible, or substitute alternative drugs for those in scarce supply. In extreme cases, the treatments are shortened to the point of ineffectiveness, and the alternative drugs used are inappropriate.

1.7 **Suppression or distortion of demand** may occur where there are marked differences between the pattern of morbidity in the community and that treated by the health facilities; inadequate or inappropriate drug supplies are often among the reasons. An overall shortage of drugs discourages patients from seeking care and suppresses overall demand, whereas plentiful supplies encourage it. If only certain drugs are in short supply, then patients are less likely to seek care when they have health problems for which these drugs would normally be used, and so the overall pattern of demand is distorted.

EXERCISE 2.A

1. Write a short explanation of the method used in your country or region to quantify drug requirements.

2. Write a short memorandum indicating whether and to what extent any of the above problems affects drug supplies in your country or region, and give what you consider to be the main reason or reasons for each problem.

MODULE 3: PREPARING AN ACTION PLAN

1. INTRODUCTION

2. TASKS IN PREPARING AN ACTION PLAN

2.A THE PREPARATORY PHASE

TASK 1:	Name the person responsible
TASK 2:	Form a working group for coordination
TASK 3:	Agree specific objectives
TASK 4:	Choose the quantification methods
TASK 5:	List tasks, estimate budget and obtain resources
TASK 6:	Programme tasks
TASK 7:	List health problems to be treated at facilities covered
TASK 8:	Select appropriate drugs for each health problem, in order to draw up essential drug list(s) for the facilities covered, and add packaging and price data
TASK 9:	Train staff in quantification methods

2.B THE QUANTIFICATION PHASE

TASKS 10-15	Data collection, quantification, costing,reconciliation to budget, calculation of final quantities per 1,000 cases
TASK 16:	Feedback results to managers for placing orders and allocating drugs to individual facilities
TASK 17:	Provide training in prescribing and stock management
TASK 18:	Evaluate the quantification process and make any necessary improvements

1. INTRODUCTION

As noted in Module 1, quantifying drug requirements is not merely an arithmetic task, and it needs to be systematically planned. It requires an **organizational structure** and **management procedures.** The **objectives** and the method or **methods** to be used must be agreed. The **physical and financial resources** needed to do the quantification must be estimated and obtained, and the **data collection and analysis** must be programmed. **Staff must be trained,** the actual **work must be managed,** and the **results must be fed back** into the drug management system **and used.** Steps must be taken to provide any **support activities** which may be necessary, such as training to improve prescribing and stock control, and finally, the effectiveness of the quantification must be **evaluated.**

The main tasks in an action plan are summarized in Table 3.1 and explained below. This module should be read quickly now to obtain a general picture of the work to be done. Do not worry if you do not understand all the details. These will become clear as you work through the succeeding modules. After you have read these, you should return to this module and read it carefully a second time.

2. TASKS IN PREPARING AN ACTION PLAN

2.A THE PREPARATORY PHASE

TASK 1: NAME THE PERSON RESPONSIBLE

- The quantification process needs a specific manager. He or she must have sufficient authority to carry through all the required activities, and must understand the methodologies being used. Normally the manager will be a senior pharmacist, medical officer, or senior administrator.

TASK 2: FORM A WORKING GROUP FOR COORDINATION

The working group should include:

Senior medical administrators and clinicians, to provide the necessary inputs on the kinds of patients to be treated at different types of facilities, to decide on essential drug lists and, if the morbidity method is used, to organize the preparation and introduction of standard treatment schedules.

Managers responsible for health information, to advise on the data available concerning patient work loads and drug use, and to plan collection of extra data if necessary. These managers may include both Ministry level epidemiologists and administrators and staff responsible for operational management at regional and unit level.

Table 3.1
Main tasks in preparing an action plan

A. Preparatory Phase

1. Name the person who will be **responsible** for the quantification. (page 3.2)

2. Form a **working group** for doordination between the parties involved: administration, finance, drugs and medical supplies, clinical services. (p. 3.2)

3. Agree the specific **objectives** of the quantification aqnd the type(s) of facilities to be covered. (p. 3.4)

4. Choose the quantification **method(s)**. (p. 3.6)

5. List **tasks** to be performed, and estimate and obtain the ecessary resources and budget (staff, transport, stationery, extra salaries and expenses etc.). (p. 3.10)

6. **Programme** tasks to be performed. (p. 3.11)

7. List **health problems to be treated** at the type(s) of facilities to be covered. (pp. 3.11, 4.1)

8. Select appropriate drugs for each health problem, in order to draw up **essential drug list(s)** for the facilities covered, and add **packaging** and **price data**. (p. 3.12)

9. **Train staff** in quantification methods, (p.1.6)

B. Quantification phase

Morbidity method	**Consumption method**
10. Draw up average standard drug **treatment schedules** for quantification (p. 5.2)	10. Select **"standard" facilities** and decide sample period (p. 8.2)
11. Tabulate number of **episodes of treatment** for each health problem. Or, if data not available, conduct a sample survey, and estimate total number of episodes of treatment (p. 6.3)	11. Estimate **total number of patient contacts** at all facilities of the type(s) concerned (p. 8.4)
12. Calculate **quantities required** of each drug (p. 7.1)	12. Calculate average drug use per 1,000 patient contacts and **quantities required** of each drug (p. 8.5)

13. Estimate **cost** of drug quantities required. (p. 7.15)

14. **Reconcile** quantities to budget if necessary. (p. 7.22)

15. Calculate **drugs required per 1,000 treatment episodes** or per 1,000 patient contacts. (p. 7.27)

16. **Feed back** results to managers for placing orders and allocating drugs to individual facilities. (p. 3.12)

17. Provide **prescribing** and **stock control** guidelines and **training**. (p. 3.12)

18. **Evaluate** the quantification **process** and **make** any necessary **improvements**. (p. 3.13)

Pharmacists, to provide technical and price information on drugs.

Finance officers, to provide information on budgetary and foreign exchange possibilities and constraints.

TASK 3: AGREE SPECIFIC OBJECTIVES

The ultimate objectives of quantifying drug requirements are to ensure that appropriate drugs are available to treat the expected case load of patients at the facilities concerned, and more broadly to promote and maintain the rational and economic use of drugs. To translate these broad objectives into operational terms a number of practical questions must be answered.

(1) **Scope: What is to be the scope of the quantification?** This decision involves three elements:

(a) **What geographical area is to be covered?** Most of the quantity estimates done so far have covered whole countries, but the methodology can be applied just as well at regional, provincial or other levels.

(b) **What health facilities and services are to be included?** Ultimately, the quantity estimates should cover all public health facilities and services. However, it is generally easier to proceed in stages. So far, countries which have introduced systematic quantification have started with primary care facilities and services, that is village health workers, health posts, health centres and preventive services, because this level of care is less complex to start with, and because it is a priority in terms of improving access to health care.

(c) **What drugs are to be included?** Quantity estimates are generally made specifically for each type of health facility or service. They should cover the agreed list of essential drugs to be provided for each type. This list should be decided before quantification begins.

(2) **Level: At what administrative level are estimates to be made?**

If there is a relatively uniform pattern of morbidity and use of health service nationally, a single national level estimate may be done. However, if there are important differences between regions, the national estimate may need to be built up by region or groups of regions with similar morbidity patterns. For example, the national estimate might be made up from one estimate for dry mountain regions and one for wet coastal ones. They may also differentiate rural and urban areas.

(3) **Special requirements: Are there any special considerations to be taken into account?** Some typical examples might be:

(a) Are the estimates intended to improve the cost-effectiveness of prescribing, or are they to be based primarily on existing prescribing patterns?

(b) Are the facilities and services whose needs are being quantified new or existing ones, and are their needs stable, or expanding or contracting?

(c) Are the estimates subject to a predetermined budget, or are they to provide the basis for drawing up a budget or for preparing a case for donor support?

(d) Are the estimates subject to predetermined foreign exchange allocations, or are they to provide a basis for negotiating them?

(e) Are there any special requirements concerning the form of the results, for example the translation of estimated drug requirements into the form of standard drug kits?

(4) Precision: What level of precision should be sought?

In principle estimates of drug requirements should be as precise as possible. However, it must be borne in mind that the level of diagnostic discrimination that may realistically be expected differs according to the skills and resources available at each type of facility. For example, staff at lower level facilities, such as health posts, may not be trained or equipped to distinguish between different types of ear infections or different skin diseases.

If the morbidity method is being used it might be tempting to do a special study to make these precise differential diagnoses, and to quantify the specific drug requirements for each one. For example, aluminium acetate drops and acetylsalicylic acid tablets might be specified for otitis externa, and procaine benzyl penicillin for otitis media.

However, if the staff delivering the care are unable to make this distinction, their practical strategy might be to treat all ear infections as otitis externa in the first place, and to give the antibiotic treatment only if there is no improvement. Then the drug quantities they actually need will be those needed to apply this trial and error strategy.

In practice, **the level of diagnostic precision used should therefore reflect the actual precision which can be achieved by the staff delivering care at the facilities concerned.**

(5) Frequency: How often should formal quantifications, using one of the two methods, be done?

Most countries work on an annual budgetary cycle, and must therefore prepare annual drug estimates. This does not mean that a formal quantification exercise is necessary every year. When formal quantification is introduced, it usually takes a few years for the drug supply system to stabilize. Once this period is over, it is often sufficient to do full-scale quantification only once every two or three years, with standard increases in intervening years to allow for demographic changes, health service developments, and any specific problems arising with particular drugs. A convenient strategy is to do a formal quantification for different types of facility each year, so that all types are re-done every three to four years. This is particularly important in order to assess the adequacy of the estimates and to update them.

EXERCISE 3.A:

> **Specify the objectives of the quantification you propose to undertake.**
>
> **The answers to this exercise will evidently vary from situation to situation, so no standard answer can be given.**

TASK 4: CHOOSE THE QUANTIFICATION METHODS

There is no single "best" way to quantify drug requirements. The method used should be chosen according to (a) the purpose for which the quantification results are to be used, (b) the actual and potential availability of the data needed for quantification, and (c) the organization of the drug supply system.

Table 3.2 compares the main advantages and disadvantages of the two principal quantification methods - the morbidity method and the consumption method.

(1) **The morbidity method:** If any of the following conditions apply, then the morbidity method may be the more appropriate method of quantifying drug requirements.

(a) Available **consumption data** are incomplete or unreliable.

(b) **Prescribing patterns** are not cost-effective, and a systematic improvement is required.

(c) The **budget** is unlikely to be sufficient to meet estimated requirements.

(d) The health facilities or services concerned are **new, or expanding or contracting rapidly**, so that past consumption is not a reliable guide to future requirements.

In theory, the morbidity method should provide a "truer" estimate of drug requirements than the consumption method. However, it is more demanding both in terms of the data required and the conditions which have to be observed by the health services:

Table 3.2
Choosing the appropriate quantification method

The patient morbidity standard treatment method	The adjusted consumption method
ADVANTAGES	
Does not require drug consumption data; useable for new services where such data are not available.	Does not require detailed morbidity data or standard treatment schedules.
Based on rational prescribing; provides a systematic basis for reviewing drug use and prescribing, especially in primary care where drug treatments are fewer and simpler.	Requires less detailed calculations.
Motivates reliable morbidity recording.	Useful for facilities like hospitals where health problems are numerous and drug treatments complex.
	Reliable if consumption is well-recorded and stable, and not likely to differ widely from current supply.
	Identifies stock management problems and encourages improvements.
DISADVANTAGES	
Detailed morbidity data and agreed standard treatment schedules may both present difficulty.	Reliable drug consumption data may be difficult to obtain especially in new or rapidly changing services.
Requires more detailed calculations.	Does not provide a detailed and systematic basis for reviewing drug use and improving prescribing; if prescribing is poor and not corrected, this method may perpetuate it.
Results may differ significantly from actual drug supply.	
Supply will not match use if standard treatments are not observed.	Unreliable if there have been long stock-outs (over 3 months), high drug wastage or losses.
Estimates only the quantitites needed to dispense to patients; separate allowances are needed for wastage and losses.	Does not encourage good morbidity recording.

(a) **Accurate morbidity profiles** are needed, giving the number of patients expected to require treatment for each health problem at the type(s) of facilities or services whose drug needs are being quantified. When such data is available, it is often incomplete or inaccurate or both. If it is not available, then it can be time-consuming, difficult, and costly to collect. If inaccurate estimates are used, they can cause serious errors in the estimated drug quantities.

(b) The process of **drafting standard drug treatment schedules based on average doses**, for quantification purposes, (called average standard treatment schedules for short) can be time-consuming, particularly at hospital level, where there is a larger variety of health problems and drug treatments are more complex.

(c) It is not sufficient to achieve agreement within the group drafting the average treatments. **Standard treatment schedules must be accepted by prescribers and adhered to in practice.** In other words, though the treatment of individual cases will vary according to clinical criteria, the **average** treatment given for a given health problem must follow what is specified in the average treatment schedule.

If average prescribing practice differs significantly from what has been specified in the average schedules, then there will be major discrepancies between the drugs supplied and those used, and shortages and surpluses will occur which would probably not have occurred with the consumption method.

However, if the specified average treatments represent an important improvement in the standard of prescribing, such discrepancies may be considered an acceptable short-term price to pay for more rational prescribing in the medium and long term.

(2) **The consumption method:** In adequately funded and well established drug supply systems, with good stock control, reliable distribution, and rational prescribing, drug requirements are usually based on projections from past consumption. If errors are made, for example because a new drug replaces an old one, or is much more heavily used than anticipated, such systems are close enough to suppliers and well enough organized to correct such errors quickly.

The consumption method may be preferred if the following conditions can be satisfied:

(a) **Accurate consumption data are available** or reasonably easily obtainable.

(b) The consumption method estimates drug requirements on the basis of actual drug use per thousand patients in a sample of "standard" facilities where the **pattern of morbidity treated is considered reasonably representative for facilities of the type or types concerned,** and the **types and quantities of drugs prescribed are considered appropriate**. There must therefore be a **sufficient number of "standard" facilities** which meet these criteria of representative morbidity and acceptable prescribing. Otherwise, the estimate will be based on atypical morbidity patterns or irrational prescribing practices or both, and drug supplies will be inappropriate.

(c) **Drug supplies at the "standard" facilities have been adequate** (in practice, essential drugs have not been out of stock for more than three months in the year). If drug shortages were too extensive, it is very difficult to estimate what drug consumption might have been if supplies had been adequate.

(d) **Stock management** is reasonably good, and wastage and losses through date expiry, damage, and theft, are not excessive.

Criteria (a) and (b) mean that the consumption method is difficult to use or inappropriate for new services, or for services expanding or contracting rapidly.

If these conditions are met, the consumption method is fast, requires less data and calculation, and the quantities estimated are less likely to differ widely from the drug quantities already being supplied.

(3) **Matching the method to the situation:** In summary, it can be seen that neither of the two methods is always better; they simply suit different conditions and objectives.

The **morbidity method** is generally better for new or rapidly changing services, or where services are being substantially reorganized. It is also better if prescribing practices are expensive and irrational because it provides a systematic basis for improvement. Finally, it is well adapted to the development of the kit system of drug supply.

The **consumption method** is generally better in the opposite circumstances. That is, for stable programmes where funding, drug management, and prescribing are reasonably good. It is also easier to use in facilities like hospitals where there is a greater variety of health problems and treatments are more complex.

In practice, the most effective approach may well be to use the two methods in combination. For example, initial estimates might be made by the morbidity method, to establish a base from which to start, and once this is assured the consumption method might be used. Alternatively, the consumption method might be used first to improve quantification in the short run and then the morbidity method might be applied progressively for each type of facility or service, so that prescribing standards can be reviewed and improved.

EXERCISE 3.B

1. For each of the two quantification methods make a list or table of:

   (a) The data required and its availability in your health system
   (b) The likely advantages of each method for your needs
   (c) The likely disadvantages of each method for your needs

2. Based on the objectives you decided in exercise 3.A, and the answers you have given to the above questions, choose the quantification method which is best suited to your needs and circumstances.

3. Describe how you might combine the two methods, and what you might gain from such a combined approach.

This exercise should be done now and reviewed after you have worked through Modules II and III. The purpose of the exercise is to enable you to make an initial assessment of the quantification method best suited to your own needs and data. No standard answer can therefore be given.

TASK 5: LIST TASKS, ESTIMATE BUDGET AND OBTAIN RESOURCES

The main tasks involved in quantification were listed in Table 3.1. In principle, quantification is part of the normal work of the drug management system and will be done by health service staff. However, if it is being done formally for the first time, there will be a certain number of additional activities for which particular resources and budget may be needed. For example, the travelling and subsistence expenses of the working group need to be covered. If the morbidity method is used, the expenses of the group charged with preparing the average standard drug treatment schedules for quantifying requirements must also be covered. If routine consumption data have to be assembled from scattered "standard" facilities, or a sample patient morbidity survey is needed, these too are likely to require additional resources and budget, or at least the permission to use those already available.

EXERCISE 3.C

As you work your way through the succeeding modules of the manual, estimate the resources and budget needed for each task.

TASK 6: PROGRAMME TASKS

It is important to programme the various tasks; first, to see wnen the necessary resources will be needed and to ensure they are available, and second, to ensure that the various tasks are sequenced in a logical order and coordinated. An agreed programme also helps ensure that the results will be available at the appropriate times for use in the drug supply planning system.

A simple visual device for summarizing your programme is a control chart. The time scale is shown across the top, and each task is shown in the form of a bar indicating its starting time, duration, and completion time. Dependencies between tasks, where a particular task can only begin when certain preceding one(s) have been completed, can be shown by dotted lines between the tasks concerned.

As far as the actual management of the programme is concerned, two aspects may be distinguished: the management of the work - ensuring that tasks are carried out according to the programme; and technical supervision to resolve problems promptly and ensure that the data collection and calculations are properly done.

The management aspect is relatively straightforward. The agreed work programme as presented in the programme control chart indicates when each task or step should begin, its duration and its finishing time.

The technical control and supervision may be somewhat more demanding. The main requirements here are that the manager of the quantification process, or a senior member of the team, should periodically check the data collection activities and the subsequent calculations, and be available should the more junior staff require advice in case of difficulty.

The details of preparing average standard drug treatment schedules are dealt with in Module 5.

EXERCISE 3.D

As you work your way through the succeeding modules of the manual, programme the various tasks in a bar chart.

TASK 7: LIST HEALTH PROBLEMS TO BE TREATED AT FACILITIES COVERED

Deciding what health problems are to be treated at the type(s) of facilities to be included in the quantification is a matter of health policy which extends far beyond quantification of drugs. The relevance of these decisions for quantification is that they are an important preparatory step before essential drug lists can be drawn up or, if lists are already available, before they can be reviewed. The drugs to be provided will depend on the health problems which each type of facility is considered capable of diagnosing and treating. These decisions are also the starting point for the preparation of the average standard drug treatments needed in the morbidity method.

The procedure for this task is described in Module 4.

TASK 8: SELECT APPROPRIATE DRUGS FOR EACH HEALTH PROBLEM, IN ORDER TO DRAW UP ESSENTIAL DRUG LIST(S) FOR THE FACILITIES COVERED, AND ADD PACKAGING AND PRICE DATA

The procedure for this is explained in Module 4.

TASK 9: TRAIN STAFF IN QUANTIFICATION METHODS

An indicative schedule for a training course has already been given in Module 1.

2.B THE QUANTIFICATION PHASE

TASKS 10-15: DATA COLLECTION, QUANTIFICATION, COSTING, RECONCILIATION TO BUDGET, CALCULATION OF FINAL QUANTITIES PER 1,000 CASES

These tasks, concerning data collection, calculation procedures, costing, reconciling estimated quantities to fit the budget (if necessary), and calculating final drug quantities per 1,000 cases (for allocating drugs to individual facilities) are explained in detail in Modules 5-8.

TASK 16: FEED BACK RESULTS TO MANAGERS FOR PLACING ORDERS AND ALLOCATING DRUGS TO INDIVIDUAL FACILITIES

The quantification will be effective only if its results are fed back to the managers of the drug supply system in a timely and convenient manner. Results that are to be used for making drug orders should be ready in time to be used in the budgeting and ordering cycle. Similarly, if the estimates are to be used to decide the quantities of drugs to be allocated to individual facilities, they should be made available to the distribution centres and to the facilities themselves well in advance.

TASK 17: PROVIDE TRAINING IN PRESCRIBING AND STOCK MANAGEMENT

Both quantification methods use "standards" of good prescribing. The morbidity method specifically defines average quantities of drugs required per standard treatment, for each health problem. The consumption method does so implicitly, by basing the quantification on the consumption patterns of "standard" facilities where prescribing is considered to be acceptable.

It is therefore important to ensure that prescribers in the facilities covered by the quantification process base their prescribing on the average standard treatments that have been used to quantify requirements. Otherwise, the drugs supplied will be based on rational standards while prescribing will continue much as before, and shortages and surpluses will continue to occur.

A number of methods may be used to improve prescribing and stock management:

(a) **Dissemination of the average standard treatment schedules used for quantifying requirements (if the morbidity method is used).** The schedules should be accompanied by a short clear explanation of the basic concept of standard treatment schedules. (These are explained in Module 5). This material should be distributed to prescribers in all the facilities covered by the quantification process.

(b) **Dissemination of clinical drug treatment schedules.** As will be explained in more detail in Module 5, the standard treatment schedules used for quantification purposes give only the average quantities of each drug required for a standard course of treatment of each health problem. They do not indicate what should be given to individual patients. In other words, they are not clinical treatment schedules. However, once quantification schedules have been established, clinical schedules can progressively be developed from them, and distributed to prescribers in the form of therapy notes, building up to a therapy manual.

(c) **Wall charts are also a good vehicle for summarizing drug treatment schedules.** They are a valuable support to information provided in manuals, for they can be consulted at a glance, and ensure that all health workers are constantly reminded of the treatment standards to apply.

(d) **The above three written aids should be supported by training seminars,** particularly for primary health care workers, but also for doctors, to explain how the standard treatments have been developed and updated, and why the guidelines should be followed.

(e) **Therapeutic consensus groups** may also be useful. These are groups where experts present and discuss standard treatment guidelines with prescribers, in order to arrive at an agreed treatment policy.

(f) **Monitoring of prescribing patterns** is another important support activity in improving prescribing. Supervising medical staff should check, during their supportive visits of inspection, whether the recommended drug treatment schedules are being observed, and find out the reasons for any important deviations.

(g) **Training in the basic principles of stock management.** It is important to keep simple stock records and to observe proper storage and security rules, e.g. the "first in first out" rule.

TASK 18: EVALUATE THE QUANTIFICATION PROCESS AND MAKE ANY NECESSARY IMPROVEMENTS

The ultimate objectives of quantifying drug requirements are to ensure that appropriate drugs are available to treat the expected case load at each health facility, and, more broadly, to promote the rational and economic use of drugs.

However, the extent to which these ultimate objectives are achieved cannot be used to evaluate the effectiveness of quantification. For, as noted in Module 1, quantification is only one component in the drug management system. All the others (selection, procurement and quality control, distribution and storage, prescription and use) have also to be carried out effectively to achieve the ultimate objectives noted above.

We must therefore fall back on evaluating the effectiveness with which the various tasks in the quantification process have been carried out. These tasks are conveniently summarized in the objectives of the manual itself in Module 1, and they are used here as evaluation criteria

Objective 1. Assess the need for more systematic quantification.

At a minimum this assessment may only result in the decision that more systematic quantification is needed. Thoroughly done, it provides a valuable diagnosis of the priority problem areas, such as irrational prescribing, or the type of facilities most in need of better quantification. This diagnosis in turn provides a sound base on which to set specific practical objectives for the quantification.

Objective 2. Set specific practical objectives for the estimates to be made.

The two basic questions here are:

(a) Did the objectives set cover the priority problems?

(b) Were the objectives sufficiently clear to avoid confusion during the actual work?

Objective 3. Choose the most appropriate method(s) to use.

The evaluation here revolves around the following questions:

(a) Did the quantification method or methods chosen allow the objectives set to be satisfied?

(b) If there have been difficulties, would a different choice of method(s) resolve them, or are other changes needed, for example, better data collection?

Objective 4. Decide what health problems are to be treated at different types of facilities.

Deciding what health problems may be treated at different types of facilities is an important preparatory step before essential drug lists can be drawn up or reviewed for these facilities, and before average standard treatments can be decided - if the morbidity method is used. As already noted, such decisions are matters of health service policy, extending far beyond the quantification of drug requirements. The key criteria in making these decisions are, on one hand the pattern of morbidity to be treated, and on the other, the diagnostic and therapeutic capabilities available at each type of facility.

The actual quantification process will not provide much new information on the appropriateness of the decisions taken, but the experience of staff actually delivering care should be monitored to see whether there are any unforeseen effects. For example, staff at some levels may be less capable than was thought at diagnosing certain conditions or using certain drugs, which may lead to indiscriminate prescribing. On the other hand, a decision that certain health problems may be treated only at higher level health facilities may cause delay in treatment if patients are reluctant to travel to these facilities.

Objective 5. Prepare or review essential drug lists.

This task is strictly speaking part of drug selection and not of quantification, but again it is too important an input of quantification to be taken for granted. It is explained in some detail in Module 4 and is worth evaluating along with the quantification process.

In principle, the effectiveness with which this task has been done can be evaluated by reference to the criteria for selecting essential drugs (listed in Module 4, Table 4.4).

Three questions should be asked here:

(a) Do any of the drugs selected fall seriously short of these criteria?

(b) Have the lists been found adequate to meet patient needs?

(c) Have the staff been able to use the drugs appropriately, and if not, what changes might be envisaged in the essential drug list or lists concerned?

Objective 6. Prepare or review standard drug treatment schedules for quantification purposes based on average doses (morbidity method only).

The procedure for this task is explained in detail in Module 5. The criteria for deciding average standard treatment schedules are essentially the same as the criteria for selecting essential drugs (as listed in Module 4, Table 4.4), supplemented by guidance from experienced clinicians on the most appropriate average treatment schedule (that is, the most suitable dosage form and strength of the drug, the average dose, the average number of times it should be given daily, and the average number of days during which treatment should be continued).

Four questions should be answered here:

(a) Do the average treatment schedules meet the criteria in Table 4.4?

(b) Are there any objections to the schedules on clinical grounds? For example, that doses are too high or too low or that treatment should be longer or shorter?

(c) Are there any objections to the schedules for practical, logistical, or cultural reasons? For example, a course of six hourly injections for two days might be the ideal treatment clinically for a particular disease, but it is not at all well adapted for ambulatory treatment, especially if patients have to travel substantial distances to come for treatment. Similarly, a pessary or a suppository might be clinically ideal for certain conditions, but unfamiliar or culturally objectionable to the patients.

(d) The final question is, once again, what has been the practical experience with these average treatment schedules? This question, however, goes beyond the adequacy of the schedules themselves, and includes issues of communication and training as discussed in task 17 above. The key sub-questions here are therefore:

d.1 Have the average treatment schedules been published and given to the prescribers?

d.2 Have the schedules been understood - are they accompanied by adequate training and explanation?

d.3 Have the schedules been accepted and applied - if not what are the reasons?

Objective 7. Collect morbidity and drug use data from routine sources, or where necessary through special estimates.

The most practical and useful way to evaluate the quality of data and the effectiveness of collection is to keep a fairly detailed record of what was done, and the problems encountered. For each type of data five questions might be asked:

(a) Were the data available - or did they have to be collected specially?

(b) Were the data complete - if there were gaps, what were they and why did they arise?

(c) Were the data reliable - if not, what aspects posed problems and why?

(d) Were the data detailed enough for quantification purposes - if not, what aspects were not and how were the problems resolved?

(e) What steps have been taken to improve the completeness and the quality of data?

Objectives 8 and 9. Calculate future drug quantities needed and cost them.

Here again it is quite useful to record how the calculations were done and the problems encountered. In keeping this record three questions should be particularly kept in mind:

(a) Were any errors made systematically or repeatedly? If so then the training was probably inadequate on these points.

(b) Were any changes made in the calculation procedures? If so, why were they needed and were they successful?

(c) It is often important to know what proportion of costs have to be paid in foreign exchange. Has this proportion been calculated?

Objective 10. Plan budget allocations and reconcile estimate quantities to fit available budget.

The main issues here are:

(a) Was the actual budget significantly lower than the budget estimated to be needed, and if so, was a sound case presented for an increase? If such a case was made why was it not accepted, and what are the implications? For example, would it be justified to cut other items within the health budget in order to increase the drug budget? Are prescription charges or other fees a feasible source of extra funding?

(b) If the estimated quantities had to be reduced to fit within available budget, were the reductions made on the basis of the priority allocated to each drug?

Objective 11. Use the final estimates to order drugs from suppliers and to issue them to health facilities.

The question here is straightforward - were the estimates used to order and issue drugs? If not, why not? If so, were the users satisfied with the information or do they want changes made, such as different timing, or different presentation?

Objectives 12 and 13. Evaluate the effectiveness of the quantification and refine estimates in successive periods.

The evaluation should include a self-check on its own adequacy.

(a) Were all aspects evaluated?

(b) Have the causes of all the main problems been identified?

(c) Have appropriate solutions been found to these problems?

(d) Are the estimates sufficiently accurate or do they need to be refined and, if so, have the necessary modifications been introduced particularly concerning improvements in the data?

Objective 14. Incorporate the quantification procedure into the routine management procedures of the drug supply system.

When formal quantification procedures are first introduced, there is often external technical and financial support which gives them a certain impetus. It is important to ensure that the procedures become part of the standard management routines as early as possible. Otherwise, they may all too easily fall into disuse. The question during evaluation is therefore whether this integration has been done.

(a) Who is responsible for quantification?

(b) Is there a definite programme cycle?

(c) Are the necessary resources and budget allowed for?

MODULE 4:

DRAWING UP AND REVIEWING ESSENTIAL DRUG LISTS BY TYPE OF FACILITY

1. INTRODUCTION

Tasks 1 – 6 from Table 3.1 have been discussed in Module 3. As noted in Module 1 section 1, the selection of drugs is a prior and separate procedure to the quantification procedure dealt with in this manual. The two quantification methods explained in Parts II and III below assume that the essential drug lists have been selected for each type of facility. However, for reference, the selection procedure for drawing up essential drug lists by type of facility is explained and illustrated in section 2 below.

2. TASK 7 – 8: DECIDING LEVELS OF CARE AND ESSENTIAL DRUG LISTS BY TYPE OF FACILITY

Drawing up an essential drug list for a given level of care or a particular type of facility involves two basic decisions: what health problems are to be treated (rather than being referred to a higher level) and what drugs are to be used to treat these health problems? The steps involved are summarized in Table 4.1, then explained and illustrated.

Table 4.1
Summary of steps in deciding levels of care and essential drug lists by facility

Step	Procedure
1.	List the major health problems encountered in the country/region concerned.
2.	Decide which health problems may be treated by each type of facility.
3.	Choose the essential drugs considered appropriate to treat/prevent the above health problems, following the criteria in Table 4.4.
4.	List the drugs alphabetically and by therapeutic group.

STEP 1: LIST THE MAJOR SPECIFIC HEALTH PROBLEMS ENCOUNTERED IN THE COUNTRY OR REGION CONCERNED

If patient morbidity statistics are not recorded, the simplest basis from which to start is the WHO International Classification of Diseases, or some derivative of it. This does not mean that the full detail of the ICD coding should be used, for it would imply extremely detailed differential diagnoses. In principle, the health problems should be defined according to the level of diagnostic discrimination which may realistically be expected at each level or type of health facility. However, if patient morbidity statistics are recorded it is usually more convenient to use the same basis for the health problems list.

EXAMPLE:

Table 4.2 shows an illustrative health problem list for community or village health workers, representing the first level of care, and health centres representing the middle level of care. The health problems are listed following the sequence of the International Classification of Diseases (ICD) in column 2 and the ICD code numbers of the conditions included in each health problem are given in column 1. Problems which would need to be referred to a higher level than the health centre have been omitted for simplicity. Columns 3 and 4 are explained in step 2 below.

STEP 2: DECIDE WHICH HEALTH PROBLEMS MAY BE TREATED AT EACH TYPE OF HEALTH FACILITY

These decisions mean looking at the diagnostic and prescribing capabilities available at each level, and deciding for each health problem whether they are sufficient to allow treatment to be provided. The range of conditions which may be treated will increase with the level of care. For example, at the community health worker level only a limited number of conditions will be treatable. At the health centre level a considerably larger range will be treatable, and so on through successive levels of care to the referral hospital level.

The treatment considered possible and desirable may be a complete treatment, or an initial treatment to help control the health problem while the patient is referred to a higher level of care. It may also be a follow-up treatment prescribed and supervised by a higher level of care to be given by a lower level facility, for example, anti-hypertensive drugs decided by a hospital specialist but delivered long term by a health centre.

EXAMPLE:

Columns 3 and 4 of Table 4.2 show an illustrative allocation of health problems between two levels of care: community health workers (CHW) and health centres. The level or levels at which it is considered a health problem may be treated are shown by a letter in the appropriate column or columns. The letters used give additional information about each health problem:

X: *Health problems for which drug treatments are indicated.*

C: *Chronic health problems; these may initially have been referred to a higher level or diagnosis but whose treatment can be delivered under supervision at a lower level.*

R: *Repeat visits for treatment of a problem diagnosed at a first visit (injections, dressings, and medication, follow-up).*

S: *Preventive health services such as vaccinations and immunizations or antenatal care.*

Of the 94 health problems included in the illustrative list, it can be seen that 81 are acute, 8 are chronic, and 5 are preventive. The remaining 4 items are repeat visits for treatment. All 94 health problems may be treated at the health centre level, but only 29 may be treated by CHWs. (24 acute, no chronic, and 5 preventive). For example, acute diarrhoea (code 009.2) may be treated at both levels, but bacillary dysentery may be treated only at the health centre.

It is emphasized that these allocations are purely illustrative, and each country must decide its own, according to its health problems and health service capabilities at each level of care. Table 4.3 shows the CHW listing separately.

EXERCISE 4.A

Read through Table 4.2

1. Taking account of the circumstances in your own country, decide what problems should be treated:

   (a) at the health centre (middle) level,

   (b) at the community health worker level

2. Add any problems you wish to include and decide at what level(s) they should be treated.

Table 4.2
Illustrative health problem listing for surveying drug requirements for the first level (community health worker) and the middle level (health centre)

Int.Clss Disease ICD code		Comm. Hlth.W. (CHW)	Middle Level (H.Centre)
	KEY:		
X	Health problems with drug requirements	24	81
C	Chronic health problems, if necessary with supervision from higher level	-	8
R	Repeat visit for same health problem	4	4
S	Health services provided	5	5
NEC	Not elsewhere classified		
	I. INFECTIOUS AND PARASITIC DISEASES		
	Bacterial infections and zoonoses		
001	Cholera		X
002.0	Typhoid		X
004	Bacillary dysentery		X
009.2	Acute diarrhoea	X	X
011	Pulmonary tuberculosis		C
030	Leprosy		C
	Other bacterial infections and zoonoses		
	Viral and chlamydial infections		
052	Chickenpox		X
055	Measles		X
076	Trachoma		X
	Other viral and chlamydial infections		
	Malaria		
084	Malaria	X	X
	Venereal diseases		
090-7	Syphilis		X
098.0	Gonorrhoea		X
098.4	Ophthalmia neonatorum		X
	Other venereal diseases		
	Fungal infections		
110	Fungal skin infections		X
112.1	Candidiasis, vaginal		X
	Other fungal infections		
	Helminthic infections		
120.0	Schistosomiasis Haematobia		X
120.1	Schistosomiasis Mansoni		X
120.2	Schistosomiasis Japonica		X
123.3	Taeniasis (tapeworm)		X
125.3	Onchocerciasis (river blindness)		X
125	Other filaria		X
126	Ancylostomiasis (hookworm)		X
127.0	Ascariasis (roundworm)	X	X
	Other helmintic infections		
	Other parasitic infections		
131.0	Trichomoniasis, vaginal		X
132	Pediculosis (lice)	X	X
133.0	Scabies	X	X
	Other parasitic infections		
	III. ENDOCRINE, NUTRITIONAL AND METABOLIC DISORDERS		
250	Diabetes mellitus		C
260-3	Malnutrition		X
264	Vitamin A deficiency, xerophthalmia		X
265-9	Other vitamin deficiency		X
	Other endocr. nutr. and metab. disorders		
	IV. DISEASES OF BLOOD AND BLOODFORMING ORGANS		
280	Iron deficiency anaemia	X	X
282.5	Sickle cell disease		X
	Other diseases of blood and blf.organs		

continued

Table 4.2 (continued)

Int.Clss Disease ICD code		Comm. Hlth.W. (CHW)	Middle Level (H.Centre)
	V. MENTAL DISORDERS		
290-9	Psychosis		C
300.0	Anxiety neurosis		X
300.4	Depressive neurosis		X
	Other mental disorders		
	VI. DISEASES OF THE NERVOUS SYSTEM AND SENSE ORGANS		
345	Epilepsy		C
372.0	Conjunctivitis	X	X
380.1	Otitis externa		X
381-2	Otitis media		X
	Other diseases of NS and sense organs		
	VII. DISEASES OF THE CIRCULATORY SYSTEM		
390-8	Rheumatic heart disease		C
401-5	Hypertension		C
410-4	Ischaemic heart disease		X
455	Haemorrhoids		X
459.0	Shock		X
	Other diseases of circulatory system		
	VIII. DISEASES OF THE RESPIRATORY SYSTEM		
460	Common cold	X	X
463	Tonsillitis		X
465	Acute bronchitis		X
480-6	Pneumonia		X
493	Asthma		X
	Other diseases of the respiratory system		
	IX. DISEASES OF THE DIGESTIVE SYSTEM		
521.0	Caries, toothache	X	X
522.5	Dental abscess		X
528	Mouth sores		X
535-6	Gastritis, heartburn, indigestion	X	X
564.0	Constipation	X	X
	Other diseases of the digestive system		
	X. DISEASES OF THE GENITO-URINARY SYSTEM		
595	Cystitis	X	X
614	Pelvic inflammatory disease		X
	Other diseases of gen.-urinary system		
	XI. COMPLICATIONS OF PREGNANCY, CHILDBIRTH AND PUERPERIUM		
634-8	Abortion		X
650	Normal delivery		X
660-5	Abnormal delivery		X
666	Postpartum haemorrhage		X
670	Major puerperal infection		X
675	Mastitis, breast abscess		X
	Other complications		
	XII. DISEASES OF THE SKIN AND SUBCUTANEOUS TISSUE		
680-2	Boil, abcess	X	X
684	Impetigo, bacterial skin infection	X	X
691.8	Eczema		X
692	Skin allergy		X
698	Itching		X
707.9	Chronic ulcer, tropical ulcer		C
	Other diseases of the skin		
	XIII. DISEASES OF THE MUSCULOSKELETAL SYSTEM AND CONNECTIVE TISSUE		
714-6	Arthritis and arthrosis	X	X
724	Backpain, lumbago	X	X
728.0	Pyomyositis		X
	Other diseases of the MS system		

continued

Table 4.2 (continued)

Int. Clss Disease ICD code		Comm. Hlth. W. (CHW)	Middle Level (H. Centr)
	XVI. SYMPTOMS, SIGNS AND ILL-DEFINED CONDITIONS		
780.3	Convulsions, febrile		X
780.5	Insomnia		X
780.6	Fever NEC	X	X
780.7	Malaise, fatigue NEC	X	X
784.0	Headache NEC	X	X
786.2	Cough NEC	X	X
787.0	Vomiting		X
788.0	Renal colic		X
789.0	Abdominal pain NEC	X	X
789.5	Ascites		
	XVII. INJURY AND POISONING		
800-29	Fractures		X
830-9	Dislocations		X
840-8	Sprains and strains	X	X
850-4	Intracranial injury, concussion		
870-90	Open wound, laceration, major cut		X
879.9	Complicated open wound, animal or human bite		X
910-19	Superficial injury, bruise, minor cut	X	X
930	Foreign body in eye		X
940-9	Burns	X	X
960-79	Poisoning		X
989.5	Snake bite, other stings and bites		X
995.0	Anaphylactic shock		X
	Other injury or poisoning		
	REPEAT VISITS FOR SAME HEALTH PROBLEMS		
	Injections	R	R
	Dressings	R	R
	Oral medication	R	R
	Follow-up visit	R	R
	OTHER HEALTH SERVICE CONTACTS		
V03-06	Vaccinations	S	S
V20	Under-five preventive care	S	S
V22-3	Antenatal care	S	S
V25	Family planning, contraception	S	S
V70	Medical examination, no illness	S	S

Table 4.3 Illustrative health problem listing for the village health worker level (abstracted from column 3 of Table 4.2)

Int.Clss Disease ICD code		Comm. Hlth.W. (VHW)
	KEY:	
X	Health problems with drug requirements	24
R	Repeat visit for same health problem	4
S	Health services provided	5
NEC	Not elsewhere classified	
009.2	Acute diarrhoea	X
084	Malaria	X
127.0	Ascariasis (roundworm)	X
132	Pediculosis (lice)	X
133.0	Scabies	X
280	Iron deficiency anaemia	X
372.0	Conjunctivitis	X
460	Common cold	X
521.0	Caries, toothache	X
535-6	Gastritis, heartburn, indigestion	X
564.0	Constipation	X
595	Cystitis	X
680-2	Boil, abcess	X
684	Impetigo, bacterial skin infection	X
714-6	Arthritis and arthrosis	X
724	Backpain, lumbago	X
780.6	Fever NEC	X
780.7	Malaise, fatigue NEC	X
784.0	Headache NEC	X
786.2	Cough NEC	X
789.0	Abdominal pain NEC	X
840-8	Sprains and strains	X
910-19	Superficial injury, bruise, minor cut	X
940-9	Burns	X
	REPEAT VISITS FOR SAME HEALTH PROBLEMS	
	Injections	R
	Dressings	R
	Oral medication	R
	Follow-up visit	R
	OTHER HEALTH SERVICE CONTACTS	
V03-07	Vaccinations	S
V20	Under-five preventive care	S
V22-3	Antenatal care	S
V25	Family planning, contraception	S
V70	Medical examination, no illness	S

STEP 3: CHOOSE THE DRUGS TO BE USED FOR THE HEALTH PROBLEMS WHICH MAY BE TREATED AT EACH LEVEL

The end result of this step is an essential drug list for each type of facility. The criteria for choosing the drugs are the same as those indicated by WHO for drawing up a national essential drug list. See Table 4.4.

Table 4.4
Summary of guidelines for selecting essential drugs

1 In each country, essential drugs should be selected by a **local committee**, including members competent in clinical medicine, clinical pharmacology, and pharmacy, and health workers of the types who will use the drugs.

2. The international **generic name** of each drug should be used, if available.

3. Essential drugs should offer the widest possible **coverage** of the pattern of prevalent morbidity affecting the population for which they are intended.

4. The drugs selected should take account of the treatment **facilities** available; the availability, training and experience of **personnel; financial** resources and costs; and **demographic, genetic,** and **environmental** factors.

5. Only drugs for which sound **scientific data** on efficacy and safety are available should be selected.

6. Each drug selected must be available in a form in which **quality, bioavailability** and **stability** can be assured under expected local conditions (including e.g. storage conditions, and local diseases such as diarrhoea or liver disease, which may affect pharmacokinetic patterns).

7. When two or more drugs seem similar in the above respects, the choice between them should be based on a careful evaluation of their relative **efficacy, safety, quality, price,** and **availability**. Policy regarding **local manufacturing**, and its feasibility may also influence the choice.

8. **Cost** is a major selection criterion. Cost comparisons between drugs, and between drugs and non drug treatments, should include the total cost of treatment, and not only the drug costs.

9. Local health authorities should decide the level of **expertise** required to prescribe each drug or group of drugs, including the competence to make particular diagnoses.

10. Essential drugs should be formulated as **single compounds.** Fixed ratio combinations are justified only if they have a proven advantage in terms of therapeutic advantage, safety, compliance, and cost, compared to single compounds administered separately.

11. Essential drug lists should be **reviewed** at least annually. New drugs should be added only if they offer clear advantages over those previously selected. Drugs on the list should be removed if new information clearly shows they no longer have a favourable benefit/risk ratio, and/or that there are safer replacements (including non-drug treatment).

EXAMPLE:

Table 4.5 shows an illustrative worksheet for selecting the essential drug list for each facility (in this example a health centre).

Columns 1 and 2 show the ICD code numbers and the name of each problem to be treated. Where patients of different age (e.g. children and adults) or with different severities of the same disease require different dosage forms or drugs these are shown separately. (This is explained in Module 5).

Column 5 shows the generic name, dosage form and strength of the drug or drugs proposed for treating each health problem. (Each dosage form and strength is noted separately). The selection of drugs in this example follows the list of illustrative standard drug treatment schedules in Table 5.1.

Column 6 is for decisions. Drugs proposed and accepted are marked "yes" those rejected are marked "no".

Column 7 is for explanatory comments on the decisions.

NB.: The only decision being made is what drugs are to be used for each health problem. No decision is made concerning treatment schedules or average dosage.

In reality all the health problems would be dealt with in turn, but Table 4.5 shows illustrative data for a selection of the health problems decided to be treatable at the health centre level from Table 4.2.

In the illustrative table we see that for:

084 Severe malaria in adults - quinine injections have been preferred to chloroquine injections.

098.0 Gonorrhoea - it has been decided that spectinomycin injections are not needed since the Gonococci are still sensitive to other antiinfectives; penicillin resistant gonococci comprise under 1% of isolates.

120.0 Schistosomiasis haematobium - metrifonate tablets have been preferred to praziquantel tablets because they are cheaper.

120.2 Schistosomiasis mansoni - praziquantel tablets have been preferred to oxamniquine capsules for they can also be used to treat S. japonicum, and S. haematobium.

455 Haemorrhoids and proctitis - hydrocortisone cream has been preferred to suppositories which have low cultural acceptability.

480-6 Pneumonia - an initial injection of procaine benzylpenicillin, followed by phenoxymethylpenicillin tablets and paracetamol tablets, are considered more practical than injectable benzylpenicillin, which is widely used in hospital treatment of pneumonia but requires 6 hourly injections.

Table 4.5
Selecting appropriate drugs for each health problem (Worksheet and illustrative data for health centres)

ICD	Health problem	Severity	Age	Drugs proposed	Decision	Remarks
O84	Malaria					
		Severity 1	Adults	chloroquine tab 150 mg base	yes	
			Children	chloroquine syrup 50 mg/ml	yes	
		Severity 2	Adults	quinine inj 300 mg/ml	yes	
				chloroquine inj 200 mg/5 ml	no	quinine preferred
				quinine tabs 300 mg	yes	
			Children	quinine inj 300 mg/ml	yes	
				quinine tabs 300 mg	yes	
O98	Gonorrhoea					
		Areas with <1% penicill resistance		procaine benzylpenicillin 3MU inj	yes	
				probenecid tabs 500 mg	yes	
		Areas with >1% penicill resistance		spectinomycin inj 2 mg	no	penicillin resistant gonococci prevalent in less than 1%
120	Schistosomiasis haematobium					
			Adults and children	metrifonate tabs 100 mg	yes	
				praziquantel tabs 600 mg	no	too expensive
120.2	Schistosomiasis mansoni					
			Adults and children	praziquantel tabs 600 mg	yes	best treatment for S.mansoni: suitable for other types of schistosomiasis
455	Haemorrhoids					
			Adults	hydrocortisone ointment 1%	yes	
				antihaemorrhoid suppositories	no	low cultural acceptability; ointment more frequently used
480-6	Pneumonia					
		Severity 1	Adults	procaine benzylpenicillin inj 3 MU	yes	
				benzylpenicillin inj 1 MU	no	6-hourly injections impractical at health centres
				phenoxymethylpenicillin tabs 250 mg	yes	
			Children	sulfameth/trimethoprim tabs 400/80 mg	yes	chloramphenicol or ampicillin may be used as alternatives
		Severity 2	Adults	sulfameth/trimethoprim tabs 400/80 mg	yes	
			Children	benzylpenicillin inj 1 MU stat and refer for admission	yes	
		All categories		paracetamol tabs 500 mg	yes	

STEP 4: LIST THE DRUGS SELECTED ALPHABETICALLY AND BY THERAPEUTIC GROUP

The illustrative data in the worksheet in Table 4.5 show only a selection of health problems from Table 4.2, together with the drugs considered most appropriate to treat each one. In reality the completed worksheet would list all the health problems for the level of health care concerned and the corresponding drugs selected to treat them.

In order to translate this information into an essential drug list, all that needs to be done is to read through the complete worksheet and list the drugs that have been selected in alphabetical order. An example is shown in Table 4.6 for the health centre or middle level of care.

This list in turn may be reorganized by therapeutic category. An example is shown in Table 4.7. Each drug has been given a code number for easy reference. This is not necessary for hand calculations, but is useful if a computer is used. If you already have a coding system in your country then that should be used. The coding system used here is explained in the note to Table 4.7.

The essential drug lists for the health centre level of care given in Tables 4.5 and 4.6 are illustrative. They are **not** model or recommended lists. However, they are based on an extensive review of over 40 essential drug lists from different countries and may be used as a practical starting point for deciding your own list for middle level facilities.

EXERCISE 4.B

Review the list of health problems to be treated at the health centre level, (the result of Exercise 4.A), and decide on the selection of drugs for each health problem. At this stage it is not necessary to specify dosage and duration of treatment. Rearrange the list of selected drugs into an alphabetical list and a list according to therapeutic category. Compare your result with the model list in Tables 4.6 and 4.7.

3. ADD PACK SIZE AND PRICE PER PACK

Before we can use these lists for quantification and costing we must add two further items of information, the pack size, and the price per pack.

(a) Counting or prescribing units and order packs.

Counting or prescribing units: are the units in which drugs are counted and prescribed. They are shown in column two of Table 4.8. In principle these units are a single tablet, capsule, suppository, pessary, ampoule or vial. For liquids the counting or prescribing unit is the millilitre, and for creams it is the gram. However, some drugs are routinely prescribed in standard containers, of a specified capacity, for example a 25g tube of cream or a 100ml bottle of syrup. For such drugs the standard containers may be used as the counting or prescribing unit.

Whether the prescribing unit is a single unit or a standard container, fractions of the unit may be used for individual doses, for example half a pill or 5ml of syrup.

Order packs: are the packs in which drugs are ordered and delivered. Order pack size is usually expressed in terms of the number of counting units in a pack. Pack sizes are shown in column three of Table 4.8, for example a 1,000 tablet tin, a 10 ampoule box, a 1,000 ml bottle, a box of 10 tubes of 20g etc.

(b) The price per pack.

This should be the total price, including handling, freight and insurance per pack, quoted by the supplier for the order which will follow the quantification. If this price is not available, the last price paid plus an allowance for any expected price increase should be used. It is also useful to have a list of reference prices, such as the UNICEF price, for comparison in negotiating price reductions with suppliers.

EXAMPLE:

Table 4.8 shows the alphabetical drug list given in Table 4.6 with pack size and price per pack added for each drug and dosage form. The prices given are illustrative.

EXERCISE 4.C

Go back to the essential drug list you drew up for the health centre level of care in exercise 4.B, and add your own pack size and price per pack data for each drug and dosage form.

Table 4.6
Illustrative essential drug list (alphabetical) for middle or health centre level of care

Drug generic name	Dosage form and strength	Health problems for which indicated (ICD code)
acetylsalicylic acid	tab 300 mg	380.1 521.0 522.5 714-6 724 728 800-29 830-9 840-8 850-4 870-9 940.9
aluminium hydroxide	tab 500 mg	535-6
aluminium acetate	drp 13% ml	380.1
antivenom sera	inj IV 100 ml	989.5
ampicillin	cap 250 mg	670
benzathine benzylpenicillin	inj 2.4 IU vial (powder)	090-7 390-8
benzoic & salicylic acid	oin tube 25 mg	110
benzylbenzoate	lot 25% ml	133.0
calamine lotion	lot ml	052 698
chloramphenicol	cap 250 mg	002.0 728
chloramphenicol	inj 1 g amp (powder)	728
chlorhexidine	sol conc 5% ml	870-9 879.9 940-9 98
chloroquine	tab 150 mg base	84.00
chlorphenamine	tab 4 mg	786.2 989.5
chlorpromazine	tab 100 mg	290-9
dapsone	tab 50 mg	030
dextran 70	inj sol 6% 500 ml pack	459 666
diazepam	tab 5 mg	300 780.5
diazepam	inj 10mg/2ml amp	345.3 780.3
diethylcarbamazine	tab 50 mg	125.3 125
epinephrine	inj 1 mg/ml amp	493 995
ergometrine	inj 0.2 mg/ml amp	634-8 650 660-5 666
ferrous sulfate	tab 60 mg	280
ferrous sulfate & folic acid	tab 60 mg & 0.25 mg	V22-23
fluorescein	drps eye 1% 1 ml	930
folic acid	tab 1 mg	282.5
gentian violet	sol l	528 707.9
glibenclamide	tab 4 mg	401-5
glyceryl trinitrate	tab 25 mg	401-5
hydrochlorothiazide	tab 25 mg	401-5
imipramine	tab 25 mg	300.4
insulin zinc susp comp	inj 40 IU/ml 10 ml vial	250
ipecacuanha	syr 0.14% ml	960-79
lidocaine	inj sol 1% 50 ml vial	132
lindane	lot 1% ml	870-9
mebendazole	tab 100 mg	126 127.0
metrifonate	tab 100 mg	120.0
metronidazole	tab 200 mg	006-7 131.0 614
neomycin & bacitracin	oin 5mg & 500 IU tube 20g	684
niclosamide	tab 500 mg	123.3
nystatin	pes 100 000 IU	112.1
oral rehydration salts	pkt 1 litre	001 009.2
paracetamol	tab 500 mg	055 380.1 381.2 460
pethidine	inj 100 mg/2ml amp	788
phenobarbital	tab 50 mg	345.0 345.1
phenytoin	tab 100 mg	345.1
phenoxymethylpenicillin	tab 250 mg	381.2 463 480-6 522.5
praziquantel	tab 600 mg	120.1 120.2
probenecid	tab 500 mg	098.0
procaine benzylpenicillin	inj 3 MU vial (powder)	098.0 098.4 381.2 46[illegible]
promethazine	tab 25 mg	786.2 787
quinine	tab 300 mg	084
quinine	inj 300 mg/ml 2ml vial	084
Ringers solution	sol 500 ml	009.2
salbutamol	tab 4 mg	493
senna	tab 7.5 mg sennosides	564.0
spectinomycin	inj 2 g vial	098.0
streptomycin	inj 1 g vial	011
sulfamethoxazole & trimethoprim	tab 400 mg & 80 mg	001 004 381.2 480-6 595
suramin sodium	inj 1 g vial (powder)	125.3
tetracycline	cap 250 mg	001 491-2 514
tetracycline	oin eye 1% tube 5mg	076 098.4 930
thiacetazone & isoniazid	tab 150 mg & 300 mg	011
vitamin A (retinol)	cap 200 000 IU	264
water for injection	10 ml vial	For use with powder form injectables

Table 4.7
Illustrative essential drug list for middle or health centre level of care by therapeutic group

Abbreviations: A - Adults, C - Children, amp - ampoule, bot - bottle, cap - capsule, drp - drop, inj - injectable, lot - lotion, oi - ointment, pkt - packet, pes - pessary, sol - solution sup - suppository, syr - syrup, tab - tablet g - gram, mg - milligram, ml - millilitre, IU - international unit.

Note: A code system for each drug is needed only if you intend to use a computer for the calculations.
The coding system used in this table is a simple one based on the numbers used in the WHO essential drugs list (WHO The Use of Essential Drugs, Report of a WHO Expert Committee, Technical Report Series 722, Geneva, WHO, 1985). This list classifies essential drugs into 27 broad therapeutic groups and then sub divides these as necessary into sub-groups.The first two digits give the broad therapeutic group, and the next two digits give the sub-group. For example, anti-infectives are group 06. Within this group there are 9 sub-groups ranging from sub-group 06 10 which is antihelminthics, to sub-group 06 90 antitrypanosomals. The first four numbers are therefore therapeutic group and sub group numbers. This coding system has been extended here by numbering the drugs in the WHO essential drugs list in sequence WITHIN each sub-group. This number is given by the third pair of numbers. The fourth pair of numbers is used to show different dosage forms and strengths of the same drug. For example, within sub-group 06 10 antihelminthics, the first drug in the WHO list is mebendazole. It is coded 06 10 01. The 100 mg tablet is coded by an additional 01, which gives the code number 06 10 01 01. the second drug in this sub-group is niclosamide 100 mg tablet. It is coded 06 10 0201. The third drug is piperazine and it is numbered 06 10 03. However there are two dosage forms. The first is a 500 mg tablet, it becomes number 06 10 03 01. The second dosage form is a 500 mg/ml syrup, it becomes 06 10 03 02. NB. Though this coding system system is based on the WHO system used in the essential drugs list, it is given as an illustration of a simple coding system. It is NOT a model coding system.

Therapeutic group & drug code number	Generic name	Dosage form & strength
01 ANAESTHETICS		
01 10 General anaesthetics, oxygen		
01 20 Local anaesthetics		
01 20 02 01	lidocaine	inj 1% 50 ml vial
02 ANALGESICS ANTIPYRETICS & NON STEROIDAL ANTI-INFLAMMATORIES		
02 10 Non opioids		
02 10 01 01	acetylsalicylic acid	tab 300 mg
02 10 05 01	paracetamol	tab 500 mg
02 10 07 01	probenecid	tab 500 mg
02 20 Opioid analgesics & antagonists		
02 20 03 01	pethidine	inj 50 mg/ml 2 ml amp
03 ANTIALLERGICS		
03 00 01 01	chlorphenamine	tab 4 mg
04 ANTIDOTES AND OTHER SUBSTANCES USED IN POISONING		
04 10 General		
04 10 02 01	ipecacuanha	syr 0.14%
04 20 Specific	antivenom sera - see 19 20 sera and immunologicals	

continued

Table 4.7 (continued)

THERAPEUTIC GROUP & DRUG CODE NUMBER	GENERIC NAME	DOSAGE FORM & STRENGTH
05 ANTIEPILEPTICS		
05 00 01 01	diazepam inj 10 mg/2 ml in 2 ml amp- see group 24	
05 00 03 01	phenobarbital	tab 30 mg
05 00 03 02	phenobarbital	syr 15 mg/5ml
06 ANTIINFECTIVE DRUGS		
06 10 Antihelminthics		
06 10 01 01	mebendazole	tab 100 mg
06 10 02 01	niclosamide	tab 500 mg
06 10 03 01	piperazine	tab 500 mg
06 10 03 02	piperazine	syr 500mg/5 ml
06 20 Antiamoebic drugs		
06 20 01 01	metronidazole	tab 200 mg
06 30 Antibacterials		
06 31 Penicillins		
06 31 01 01	ampicillin	cap 250 mg
06 31 01 02	ampicillin	syr 125 mg/ml
06 31 02 01	benzathine benzylpenicillin	inj 2.4 mega IU/5ml
06 31 05 01	phenoxymethylpenicillin	tab 250 mg
06 31 05 02	phenoxymethylpenicillin	syr 250 mg/ml
06 31 06 01	procaine benzylpenicillin	inj 3 mega IU in vial
06 32 Other antibacterial drugs		
06 32 01 01	chloramphenicol	cap 250 mg
06 32 07 01	sulfadimidine	tab 500 mg
06 32 08 01	sulfamethoxazole + trimethoprim	tab 400 mg + 80 mg
06 32 10 01	tetracycline	tab 50 mg
06 33 Antileprosy drugs		
06 33 02 01	dapsone	tab 100 mg
06 34 Antituberculosis drugs		
06 34 05 01	streptomycin	inj 1 ml in vial
06 34 06 01	thioacetazone + isoniazid	tab 50 mg + 100 mg
06 40 Antifilarial drugs		
06 40 01 01	diethylcarbamazine	tab 50 mg
06 40 02 01	suramin sodium	inj 1 g in vial
06 50 Antifungal drugs		
06 50 03 01	nystatin	pes 100 000 IU
06 60 Antileishmaniasis drugs		
06 70 Antimalarial drugs		
06 70 01 01	chloroquine	tab 150 mg
06 70 01 02	chloroquine	syr 50 mg/5 ml
06 70 03 01	quinine	tab 300 mg
06 70 03 02	quinine	inj 300 mg/ml in 2ml amp
06 80 Antischistosomal drugs		
06 80 01 01	metrifonate	tab 100 mg
06 80 03 01	praziquantel	tab 600 mg
06 90 Antitrypanosomal drugs		
	suramin sodium - see 06 40 antifilarials above	

continued

Table 4.7 (continued)

THERAPEUTIC GROUP & DRUG CODE NUMBER	GENERIC NAME	DOSAGE FORM & STRENGTH
07 ANTIMIGRAINE DRUGS		
- -	- -	
08 ANTINEOPLASTICS AND IMMUNOSUPRESSIVE DRUGS		
- -	- -	
09 ANTIPARKINSONISM DRUGS		
- -	- -	
10 BLOOD - (DRUGS AFFECTING THE)		
10 10 Antianaemics		
10 10 01 02	ferrous sulfate	sol 15 mg iron equiv/ 0.6 ml 0.6 ml
10 10 02 01	folic acid	tab 1 mg
10 10 04 01	ferrous sulfate + folic acid	tab 60 mg + 0.20 mg
10 20 Anticoagulants and antagonists		
- -	- -	
11 BLOOD PRODUCTS AND SUBSTITUTES		
11 10 Plasma substitutes		
11 10 01 01	dextran 70	inj 6% sol
11 20 Plasma fractions		
- -	- -	
11 30 Plasma substitutes		
- -	- -	
12 CARDIOVASCULAR DRUGS		
12 10 Antianginal drugs		
12 10 01 01	glyceryl trinitrate	tab 0.5 mg
12 20 Antidysarrhythmic drugs		
- -	- -	
12 30 Antihypertensives		
12 30 02 01	hydrochlorothiazide	tab 50 mg
12 40 Cardiac glycosides		
- -	- -	
12 50 Drugs for shock or anaphylaxis		
12 50 02 01	epinephrine (adrenalin)	inj 1 mg/ml 1 ml amp
	dextran 70 see under 11 10 Plasma substitutes	
13 DERMATOLOGICAL DRUGS		
13 10 Antifungal drugs		
13 10 01 01	benzoic acid & salicylic acid	oin 6% & 3%
13 20 Antiinfective drugs		
13 20 02 01	neomycin & bacitracin	oin 5 mg & 500 IU 20 mg tube
13 30 Antiinflammatory drugs & antipruritic drugs		
13 30 02 01	calamine lotion	lot
13 30 03 01	hydrocortisone	oin 1% 15 mg tube
13 40 Astringent drugs		
13 40 01 01	aluminium acetate	sol 13% for dilution
13 50 Keratoplastics & keratolitic agents		
- -		
13 60 Scabicides & pediculicides		

continued

Table 4.7 (continued)

THERAPEUTIC GROUP & DRUG CODE NUMBER	GENERIC NAME	DOSAGE FORM & STRENGTH
13 60 01 01	benzyl benzoate	lot 25%
13 60 02 01	lindane	cream 1%
14 DIAGNOSTIC AGENTS		
- -	- -	
14 10 Ophthalmic drugs	fluorescein - see 21 ophthalmologicals logicals, and vitamin A - 27 Vitamins	
14 20 Radiocontrast media		
15 DISINFECTANTS		
15 00 01 01	chlorhexidine	sol 5%
15 00 02 01	gentian violet	sol 1%
16 DIURETICS	hydrochlorothiazide see 12 cardiovasculars	
17 GASTROINTESTINAL DRUGS		
17 10 Antacids and antiulcer drugs		
17 20 01 01	aluminium hydroxide	tab 500 mg.
17 20 Antiemetic drugs		
17 20 01 02	promethazine	tab 25 mg
17 20 01 02	promethazine	syr 5 mg/5 ml
17 30 Antihaemorrhoidal drugs	hydrocortisone - see under 13 30 antiinflammatory & antipruritic drugs	
17 40 Antispasmodic drugs		
- -	- -	
17 50 Cathartic drugs		
17 50 01 01	senna	tab 7.5 mg
17 60 Diarrhoea, drugs used in		
- -	- -	
17 62 Replacement solution		
17 62 01 01	oral rehydration salts	27.5 mg/l pkt
18 HORMONES		
18 10 Adrenal hormones & synthetic substitutes		
- -	- -	
18 20 Androgens		
- -	- -	
18 30 Contraceptives		
- -	- -	
18 40 Estrogens		
- -	- -	
18 50 Insulins & antidiabetic agents		
18 50 01 01	insulin zinc comp susp	inj 40 IU/ml 10 ml vial
18 50 02 01	glibenclamide	tab 5 mg
18 60 Ovulation inducers		
- -	- -	
18 70 Progestogens		
- -	- -	
18 80 Thyroid hormones & antithyroid drugs		
- -	- -	

continued

Table 4.7 (continued)

THERAPEUTIC GROUP & DRUG CODE NUMBER	GENERIC NAME	DOSAGE FORM & STRENGTH
19 IMMUNOLOGICALS		
19 10 Diagnostic agents		
- -	- -	
19 20 Sera and immunoglobins		
19 20 03 01	antivenom sera	
19 30 vaccines	covered by expanded programme of immunization	
20 PERIPHERALLY ACTING MUSCLE RELAXANTS & CHOLINESTERASE INHIBITORS		
- -	- -	
21 OPHTHALMOLOGICALS		
21 10 Antinfectives		
21 10 03 01	tetracycline eye oin	1% in 5 mg tube
21 20 Antiinflammatories		
- -	- -	
21 20 Local anaesthetics		
- -	- -	
21 40 Miotics and anti glaucoma drugs		
- -	- -	
21 50 Irridiatics		
21 50 01 01	fluorescein eye drp	1%
22 OXYTOCICS		
22 00 01 01	ergometrine	tab 0.2 mg
22 00 01 02	ergometrine	inj 0.2 mg/ml 1 ml amp
23 PERITONEAL DIALYSIS SOLUTION		
- -	- -	
24 PSYCHOTHERAPEUTICS		
24 10 02 01	chlorpromazine	tab 100 mg
24 00 02 02	chlorpromazine	syr 2 mg/ml
24 00 03 01	diazepam	tab 5 mg
	diazepam	inj 10 mg/2 ml 2 ml amp
25 RESPIRATORY TRACT DRUGS		
25 10 Antiasthmatics		
25 10 03 01	salbutamol	tab 4 mg
25 10 03 02	salbutamol	syr 2 mg/ml 1 ml amp
	see epinephrine (adrenalin) -	12 50 drugs for shock and anaphylaxis
25 20 Antitussives		
- -	- -	
26 SOLUTIONS CORRECTING WATER, ELECTROLYTE AND ACID-BASE DISTURBANCES		
26 10 Oral rehydration salts	see ORS under 17 62, replacement solution	
26 20 Parenteral		
26 20 01 01	Ringers solution (compound sodium lactate solution)	iv 500 ml
26 30 Miscellaneous		
26 30 09 01	water for injection	10 ml amp
27 Vitamins and minerals		
27 00 05 01	retinol (vitamin A)	tab 60 mg

Table 4.8
Illustrative essential drug list (alphabetical) for middle or health centre level of care,with order pack size and illustrative price

DRUG GENERIC NAME	DOSAGE FORM & STRENGTH	PACK SIZE	PRICE PER PACK ($)
acetylsalicylic acid	tab 300 mg	1000 tab tin	0.94
aluminium hydroxide	tab 500 mg	1000 tab tin	1.00
aluminium acetate	drp 13% ml	1000 ml bottle	3.00
antivenom sera	inj IV 100 ml	1 vial 100 ml	15.00
ampicillin	cap 250 mg	1000 cap tin	20.86
benzathine benzylpenicillin	inj 2.4 MU vial (powder)	2.4 MU vial	0.18
benzoic & salicylic acid	oint 6% & 3% mg	1 kg pot	3.61
benzyl benzoate	sol 25% ml	1000 ml bottle	1.57
calamine lotion	lot ml	500 ml bottle	1.28
chloramphenicol	cap 250 mg	1000 tab tin	9.80
chloramphenicol	inj 1 g amp (powder)	1 g vial	0.27
chlorhexidine	sol conc 5% ml	100 ml bottle	0.93
chloroquine	tab 150 mg base	1000 tab tin	5.95
chlorphenamine	tab 4 mg	1000 tab tin	0.88
chlorpromazine	tab 100 mg	100 tab tin	0.67
dapsone	tab 50 mg	1000 tab tin	0.66
dextran 70	inj sol 6% 500ml pack	500 ml bottle	0.14
diazepam	tab 5 mg	1000 tab tin	3.00
diazepam	inj 10mg/2ml amp	10 vial box	0.12
diethylcarbamazine	tab 50 mg	1000 tab tin	1.15
epinephrine	inj 1 mg/ml amp	10 amp box	0.37
ergometrine	inj 0.2 mg/ml amp	10 amp box	0.41
ferrous sulfate	tab 60 mg	1000 tab tin	0.82
ferrous sulfate & folic acid	tab 60 mg & 0.25 mg	1000 tab tin	0.76
fluorescein	drps eye 1% 1 ml	10 ml bottle	0.50
folic acid	tab 1 mg	1000 tab tin	0.58
gentian violet	sol ml	25 g tin (=1000 ml)	0.61
glibenclamide	tab 4 mg	1000 tab tin	1.50
glyceryl trinitrate	tab 25 mg	1000 tab tin	3.00
hydrochlorothiazide	tab 25 mg	1000 tab tin	2.18
imipramine	tab 25 mg	1000 tab tin	3.00
insulin zinc susp comp	inj 40 IU/ml 10 ml vial	10 ml vial	0.35
ipecacuanha	syr 0.14% ml	100 ml bottle	0.33
lidocaine	inj sol 1% 50 ml vial	50 ml vial	0.25
lindane	cream 1% 25 g	100 tubes	30.00
mebendazole	tab 100 mg	100 tab pack	0.61
metrifonate	tab 100 mg	1000 tab tin	10.00
metronidazole	tab 250 mg	1000 tab tin	5.39
neomycin & bacitracin	oint 5 mg &500 IU tube, 20g	20g tube	0.16
niclosamide	tab 500 mg	100 tab tin	1.41
nystatin	pes 100 000 IU	15 pess box	1.09
oral rehydration salts	pkt 1 litre	1 litre pkt	0.04
paracetamol	tab 500 mg	1000 tab tin	2.60
pethidine	inj 100 mg/2ml amp	10 amp box	1.00
phenobarbital	tab 50 mg	100 tab pack	0.36
phenytoin	tab 100 mg	100 tab pack	0.55
phenoxymethylpenicillin	tab 250 mg	1000 tab tin	7.51
praziquantel	tab 600 mg	1000 tab tin	376.47
probenecid	tab 500 mg	30 tab box	1.50
procaine benzylpenicillin	inj 3 MU vial (powder)	3 MU (3 g) vial	0.24
promethazine	tab 25 mg	100 tab bottle	0.34
quinine	tab 300 mg	100 tab tin	3.60
quinine	inj 300 mg/ml 2ml vial	10 vial box	0.88
Ringers solution	sol 500 ml	500 ml bottle	0.33
salbutamol	tab 4 mg	100 tab tin	1.92
senna	tab 7.5 mg	100 tab pack	2.55
spectinomycin	inj 2 g vial	10 vial box	1.00
streptomycin	inj 1 g vial (powder)	1g vial	0.10
sulfameth./trimethoprim	tab 400 mg & 80 mg	1000 tab tin	17.00
suramin sodium	inj 1 g vial (powder)	10 vial box	5.00
tetracycline	cap 250 mg	1000 cap tin	7.90
tetracycline	oint eye 1% tube 5 g	5 mg tube	0.07
thioacetazone & isoniazid	tab 150 mg & 300 mg	1000 tab tin	6.82
vitamin A (retinol)	cap 200 000 IU	1000 cap tin	2.00
water for injection	10 ml amp	10 ml amp	0.03

PART II

THE MORBIDITY METHOD

MODULE 5:

DATA REQUIREMENTS: STANDARD DRUG TREATMENT SCHEDULES FOR QUANTIFYING REQUIREMENTS, BASED ON AVERAGE DOSES

1. INTRODUCTION

Four basic sets of data are required for the morbidity method of quantifying drug requirements.

(1) **Essential drug lists with packaging and price data** for each type of facility whose drug requirements are being quantified.

(2) **Pharmaceutical budgets and foreign exchange allocations** actually or potentially available.

(3) **Standard drug treatment schedules for quantification purposes, based on average doses** (called average treatment schedules for short).

(4) A complete **patient morbidity profile** giving the number of treatment episodes for each health problem defined.

Items 1 and 2 are required for both methods of quantification; items 3 and 4 are specific to the morbidity method.

Item 1 was already dealt with in Module 4, and an illustrative essential drug list for the health centre level of care was given in Table 4.8, including packaging and price data.

Item 2 is the expected budget and foreign exchange allocation for drugs. These have to be obtained from the finance department of the Ministry of Health. The quantities of essential drugs estimated to be required by a formal quantification are quite likely to cost more than the expected budget. It is therefore important to know what this budget is, so that the size of the difference can be established. If the budget is fixed, then the estimated quantities of the various drugs have to be cut according to their relative priorities to bring them back within the budget.

In most developing countries a large proportion of drugs is imported. If foreign exchange is limited it is equally important to obtain information on the proportion of the budget actually or potentially available in foreign exchange, for the estimated requirements will also have to be adjusted to within foreign exchange allocations.

The rest of this module explains the concept of average standard treatment schedules, advises on how to prepare them, and provides an illustrative schedule for the health centre (middle) level of care. Module 6 deals with the collection of patient morbidity data.

2. TASK 10: STANDARD DRUG TREATMENT SCHEDULES FOR QUANTIFYING DRUG REQUIREMENTS, BASED ON AVERAGE DOSES (AVERAGE DRUG TREATMENT SCHEDULES)

The quantification methods in this manual assume that prescribing is rational. In order to assure that prescribing is actually rational in practice, standard treatment schedules should be made available to prescribers, as described in Module 3, task 17.

You will recall from Module 1 that the basic formula used in the morbidity method is:

Quantity of the drug specified for a standard course of treatment	x	Number of treatment episodes of the health problem	=	Total quantity of a drug required for a given health problem

The first element in the formula requires agreement on an average standard treatment schedule for each health problem. As this average treatment will be multiplied by the total number of treatment episodes for that particular health problem, it is necessary to define an **average** quantity per course of treatment.

Such an average treatment schedule is different from a clinical treatment schedule. Clinical schedules are intended to help clinical staff decide on the drug treatments to be given to individual patients. They must therefore specify all the nuances of diagnosis which require a variation in treatment for individual patients, including diagnosis, severity, age, body weight, general health status, drug resistance, etc. However, for quantification of drug needs the standard treatment schedule need not be so precise. For the calculations it is sufficient if agreement can be reached on an average drug treatment. It should be stressed that such an average drug treatment schedule is not specific enough to be used for clinical guidance.

Average drug treatment schedules have also to accommodate a system for specifying selection and dosage of drugs for patients of different age and disease severity, but this need not be so elaborate as in clinical treatment schedules. In general, two age groups should be distinguished (below five years, and five years and older), and the severity of the disease should only be included in the average drug treatment schedules if a more severe case would need a different drug. Examples have already been shown in Table 4.5, e.g. quinine injection for a case of severe or resistant malaria instead of chloroquine tablets for a mild case.

Average and clinical drug treatment schedules are of course related. **Average schedules are valid only if they represent the average treatments which will actually be used clinically.** For example, in Table 5.1, it has been decided that the standard treatment for iron deficiency anaemia (ICD 280) should be 84 tablets of ferrous sulfate, but if prescribers usually give 120 tablets, then the average does not reflect reality. The same applies if the average treatment schedule specifies one drug but prescribers continue to use another.

If clinical schedules already exist, average schedules should be derived from them. If clinical schedules do not exist or are not widely used, the following procedure is recommended. First a list of essential drugs should be prepared, based on diseases and complaints at the various levels of health care (see Module 4); then average drug treatment schedules should be drawn up, based on the essential drugs selected for each health problem. These schedules can be used for quantification purposes but are usually insufficiently detailed to be used as clinical treatment guidelines for prescribers. The average drug treatment schedules should then be expanded into clinical drug treatment schedules which can be disseminated to health workers and can be used for training. It must be emphasized that the drug need estimates, based on the average drug treatment schedules, can only hope to be accurate when a national policy to use the clinical schedules is being enforced and when prescribers actually follow them.

It is important that physicians and other higher level health service staff should be reassured **that average treatment schedules do not infringe on their clinical freedom to adapt the drug dosages to the needs of individual patients.** For example, in Table 5.1, the average standard treatment for a mild case of malaria in adults is ten 150 mg base tablets of chloroquine. This average allows for **and reflects variations in the courses of drug treatments prescribed for individual patients.**

3. GUIDELINES FOR DRAWING UP AVERAGE DRUG TREATMENT SCHEDULES

An average drug treatment schedule contains six items of information:

(1) The name of the **health problem**, and the **ICD** number or numbers of the diagnoses it includes.

(2) The **generic name of dosage form and strength** of each drug to be used in the treatment.

(3) The **average dose.**

(4) The **average number of doses per day.**

(5) The **average number of days** these doses are to be given.

(6) The **total average quantity** of each drug used for a **standard course of treatment**; or in the case of chronic conditions, where treatment is long term, the **total quantity usually given per prescription.** This total is obtained by multiplying the average dose by the average number of doses per day by the average number of days the doses are to be given.

Five different sets of criteria need to be borne in mind in drawing up or reviewing average treatment schedules:

(a) The criteria for **selecting essential drugs** in the first place (Module 4, Table 4.4) have already been applied, but should still be borne in mind.

(b) Next, more detailed **clinical criteria** must be applied to each health problem to determine the most appropriate average dosage form and strength of the drugs to be used, then the average dose, the number of doses per day, and the number of days of treatment.

If only these two sets of criteria are used, the result is theoretically ideal average treatment schedules. However, three further sets of criteria must be applied to ensure that the schedules are feasible in practice.

(c) The next criterion concerns the **capability** to administer treatment schedules. The diagnostic and treatment capabilities (including both staff skills and availability of diagnostic and support services) required to administer each treatment schedule should be borne in mind when selecting drugs for each type of facility.

(d) A further criterion is the **physical feasibility** of administering the proposed average treatment. A course of injections several times a day for several days may meet all the above criteria, but it is hardly appropriate for ambulatory care, especially in rural areas where patients may have to travel considerable distances to reach health facilities.

(e) Finally, there are **cultural** considerations. For example, pessaries or suppositories may be culturally unacceptable, while injections are regarded as the only really "strong treatment". Average treatments which go against cultural preferences may be far more effective or cost-effective, but they must be explained and made acceptable to prescribers and patients.

Drawing up well founded, practical and acceptable schedules is, however, only the first step. **The schedules will only be effective if prescribers are trained in their use, and actually apply them.** There should be continuous monitoring and feedback on what is actually happening.

The other aspect of drawing up or reviewing average treatment schedules, on which some guidance will be useful, concerns the practical organisation of the group which draws them up. Each country will of course do this according to its own health service structure and procedures, but a number of points should be observed.

First, the working group set up to coordinate and support the quantification process contains staff who have access to most of the necessary skills, knowledge, and experience to draw up or review average drug treatment schedules. A convenient solution would therefore be for the average treatment schedule group to be a sub-committee of the working group.

The three most important categories of participants in the committee that draws up or reviews average treatment schedules are:

(a) Experienced health service staff from the type of facility for which the treatment schedules are intended, who are familiar with diagnostic possibilities and prescribing patterns, and can advise on what is feasible in practice.

(b) Experienced senior clinicians in different fields, who can advise on the treatments which they consider most effective.

(c) Pharmacists and administrators who can point out technical requirements, such as special storage conditions and ensure that costs are also borne in mind, so that proposed treatments are not only effective but also cost-effective.

Open discussion between these three groups can also help identify training needs to improve diagnostic and prescribing capabilities.

4. ILLUSTRATIVE AVERAGE DRUG TREATMENT SCHEDULES FOR THE MIDDLE (HEALTH CENTRE) LEVEL OF CARE

It must be emphasized that these schedules are **not model or recommended schedules** and are not specific enough to be used as clinical treatment schedules. However, they have been developed after reviewing a large number of standard treatment manuals, and also take account of the views of clinicians and specialists familiar with the middle level of care in developing countries. Relevant WHO technical units have also been consulted in the development of this work.

They are included both as an illustration and as a practical starting point in working out your own average treatment schedules for middle level health care facilities, appropriate to your country's circumstances. (NB: these schedules may not be appropriate for estimating drug requirements at hospitals, where health problems may be differentiated into more specific diagnoses with corresponding standard drug treatments.)

EXERCISE 5 A

Read through the average treatment schedules in Table 5.1 and make any modifications and additions you think necessary to adapt the schedules to your own country's circumstances.

Table 5.1
Illustrative standard treatment schedules for quantification of drug requirements based on average doses

Introductory remarks

These drug treatment schedules have been developed after reviewing a large number of standard treatment manuals and consultations with people involved in health care. The advice of experts within WHO has also been sought and their comments taken into account. A list of a selection of publications consulted is given at the end of the module.

The drug treatment schedules that have been developed are intended for use in the quantification of essential drugs required, principally at the middle level of health care in developing countries. In certain instances they are unlikely to be appropriate for estimating drug requirements at hospitals.

It must be emphasized that these drug treatment schedules are not, in their present form, suitable for individual patient care. For individual patient care more detailed schedules are necessary which allow for detailed variation depending on such factors as body weight, knowledge of resistance of organisms to certain drug e.g. chloroquine.

For drug quantification purposes it is only necessary to indicate the overall quantity of drugs required and not those for individuals. Consequently drug treatment schedules are indicated for two main groups of people - children aged less than five years and adults..

In the preparation of these standard treatment schedules several assumptions have been made. The main ones are:

1. For drugs where body weight is important in estimating dosage an adult body weight of 60 kg has been used and for children 15 kg, unless otherwise stated. The actual dose for an individual patient will in many cases depend crucially upon body weight. This is particularly important for young children.

2. For recurrent urinary tract infections a 10-day course of antibiotics has been used.

3. For acute respiratory infections (including ear infections) in children, a five-day antibiotic course has been used.

4. For other conditions (except where there are specific drug guidelines e.g. typhoid fever or sexually transmitted diseases) in which antibiotics are indicated a five-day course has been used.

Table 5.1 (continued)

5. Where penicillin has been included as the antibiotic of choice allowance has usually been made for treatment episodes to begin with an intramuscular preparation.

6. Paracetamol has been included for all children; for adults acetylsalicylic acid has arbitrarily been used as an analgesic and paracetamol as an antipyretic.

7. For certain health problems an alternative drug is indicated to the one that is used as an illustration. The actual choice of drugs depends on the particular circumstances for which quantification is undertaken.

8. Where treatment of a health problem is for longer than four weeks (28 days) allowance should be made for this. The quantities shown in the last column "Amount per course of treatment" is for four weeks only.

9. While for many drugs syrups and elixirs are commercially available specifically for children, in these illustrative drug treatment schedules these have not been included. In their place tablets have been used. This is because tablets are far cheaper than syrups; less bulky to transport; far more stable particularly in warm weather, and the problems of breakages and waste are not so great. However, there might be situations where in view of improved compliance it is decided that paediatric preparations are more cost-effective.

10. For certain health problems where injectable preparations are indicated the amount per course of treatment in the last column of the table gives quantities which include part vials. When drug quantification is being carried out a decision must be taken on whether multi-dose vials are acceptable.

11. Sterile water is required to formulate many of the drugs included in these schedules. Requirements for this and other disposable items e.g. syringes, needles, etc., have not been included.

12. For certain health problems it could be argued that placebo drugs are justified. No allowance has been made for this in these schedules.

13. These average treatment schedules are designed for use in quantifying drug requirements at the mid-level e.g. clinics or health centres. It is assumed that the health workers at this level have been trained in diagnosis and appropriate use of drugs included in the schedules.

14. For certain health problems requiring drugs more than one level of severity has been indicated. The term severity has been used in two meanings:

    1. where the patient's condition is such that oral medication cannot be taken or retained or their state is considered to be immediately life threatening and

    2. where treatment with a first line therapy has not been successful.

Table 5.1A
Illustrative standard treatment for quantification of drug requirements based on average doses

ICD	INDICATION	DRUGS	DOSE	TIMES PER DAY	NO.OF DAYS	AMOUNT PER COURSE OF TREATMENT
1. INFECTIOUS AND PARASITIC DISEASES						
	Bacterial infections and zoonoses					
001	Cholera					
	Adults	Tetracycline 250 mg	2 caps	x 4	x 3	24 caps
		Oral Rehydr. Salts 1 ltras required				assume 4 sachets
	Children	Sulfameth/trim 400/80 mg	1 tab	x 2	x 3	6 tabs
		Oral Rehydr. Salts 1 ltras required				assume 3 sachets
002.0	Typhoid					
	Adults	Chloramphenicol 250 mg	3 caps	x 4	x 12	144 caps
	Children	Chloramphenicol 250 mg	1.5 caps	x 4	x 12	72 caps
	NB: Cases of typhoid should be reviewed at regular intervals					
004	Bacillary dysentery					
	Adults	Sulfameth/trim 400/80 mg	2 tabs	x 2	x 5	20 tabs
	Children	Sulfameth/trim 400/80 mg	1 tab	x 2	x 5	10 tabs
006	Amoebiasis					
	Adults	Metronidazole 250 mg	3 tabs	x 3	x 5	45 tabs
	Children	Metronidazole 250 mg	1 tab	x 2	x 3	6 tabs
007	Giardiasis					
	Adults	Metronidazole 250 mg	1 tab	x 3	x 5	15 tabs
	Children	Metronidazole 250 mg	1/2 tab	x 3	x 5	7.5 tabs
009.2	Acute diarrhoea, gastroenteritis					
	Severity 1 (no dehydration)					
	Adults	Oral Rehydr. Salts 1 ltras required				assume 2 sachets
	Children	Oral Rehydr. Salts 1 ltras required				assume 1 sachet
	Severity 2 (some dehydration)					
	Adults	Oral Rehydr. Salts 1 ltras required				assume 6 sachets
	Children	Oral Rehydr. Salts 1 ltras required				assume 2 sachets
	Severity 3 (severe dehydration)					
	Adults	Ringers infusion 500 ml	as required			assume 6000 ml
	Children	Ringers infusion 500 ml	as required			assume 1500 ml
		followed by ORS as in Severity 2, depending on status of the patient				
011	Pulmonary tuberculosis					
	Adults	Streptomycin	inj 1 gram	x 1	x 28	28 vials
		Thioacetazone/INH 150/300 mg	1 tab	x 1	x 28	28 tabs
	Children 12-24 kg	Streptomycin 20-40 mg/kg	assume 0.6 g	x 1	x 28	17 vials
		Thioacetazone/INH 150/300 mg	1/2 tab	x 1	x 28	14 tabs
	NB: Streptomycin is usually continued for two months and Thioacetazone/INH for twelve months					
	NB: Where adverse reactions to Thioacetazone/INH are high, ethambutol should be substituted					
	NB: Re-treatment of patients with proven resistance to INH should be undertaken by specialised, usually centralised control services. Frequently ethambutol and rifampicin will be needed for such cases.					
030	Leprosy					
	Starting dose					
	Adults	Dapsone 100 mg	1/4 tab once weekly for 4 weeks; then 1/2 tab once weekly for four weeks, then slowly increasing to maintenance dose			
	Maintenance dose					
	Adults	Dapsone 100 mg	1 tab daily for life (lepromatous leprosy) 1/2 tab daily for minimal five years (borderline and tuberculoid leprosy)			
	NB: In severe and/or resistant cases, provision of rifampicin and/or clofazimine should be considered.					
	Viral and chlamydial infections					
052	Chickenpox	Chlorphenamine 4 mg	1/2 tab	x 3	x 6	9 tabs
		Calamine lotion	as required			assume 50 ml
055	Measles					
	Severity 1	Paracetamol 500 mg	1/2 tab	x 4	x 2	4 tabs
	Severity 2	Procaine benzylpenicillin 3 MU	inj 0.3 MU inj IM	stat		1/10 vial
		Phenoxymethylpenicillin 250 mg	1/2 tab	x 4	x 5	10 tabs
		Paracetamol 500 mg	1/2 tab	x 4	x 4	8 tabs
076	Trachoma	Tetracycline eye ointment 1%	apply	x 1	x 60	2 tubes 5 g

continued

Table 5.1A (continued)

ICD	INDICATION	DRUGS	DOSE	TIMES PER DAY	NO.OF DAYS	AMOUNT PER COURSE OF TREATMENT
	Malaria					
084	Malaria					
	Severity 1					
	Adults	Chloroquine 150 mg base	4 tabs stat, then			
			2 tabs after 6 hours, then			
			2 tabs	x 1	x 2	10 tabs
	Children	Chloroquine 150 mg base	1 tab stat, then			
			1/2 tab after 6 hours, then			
			1/2 tab	x 1	x 2	2.5 tabs
	NB: In many countries tablets of 150 mg (100 mg base) are used, in which case the dosage schedule should be adapted					
	NB: In children the proper dosage should be based on body weight (25 mg/kg)					
	NB: In areas where there is known to be a significant frequency of chloroquine resistant P. falciparum locally appropriate drugs should be included.					
	Severity 2					
	Adults	Quinine 300 mg/ml	2 ml slow IV infusion			
		(as hydrochloride)	(repeat after 8 and 16 hours), then			6 ml
		Quinine 300 mg	2 tabs	x 3	x 6	36 tabs
	Children	Quinine 300 mg/ml	0.5 ml slow IV infusion			
		(as hydrochloride)	(repeat after 8 and 16 hours), then			1.5 ml
		Quinine 300 mg	1/2 tab	x 3	x 6	9 tabs
	Venereal diseases					
090-7	Syphilis	Benzath benzylpenicill 2.4 MU	2.4 MU inj IM	stat		1 vial
098.0	Gonorrhoea (areas with <1% penicillin resistance)	Procaine benzylpenicillin 3 MU	4.5 MU inj IM	stat		1.5 vial
		Probenecid 500 mg	2 tabs	stat		2 tabs
	Gonorrhoea (areas with >1% penicillin resistance)	Spectinomycin 2 gram	2 gram inj IM	stat		1 vial
	NB: Allowance should be made for drugs to treat contacts					
098.4	Ophthalmia neonatorum	Tetracycline eye ointment 1%	apply	x 24	x 1	
			then	x 8	x 1	
			then	x 4	x 8	2 tubes 5 g
		Procaine benzylpenicillin 3 MU	75000 IU inj IM	x 2	x 3	assume 1/2 vial
	Fungal infections					
110	Fungal skin infections	Benzoic & Salicylic acid ointm	apply	x 3	x 10	tube 40 gram
112.1	Candidiasis, vaginal	Nystatin pessary 100 000 IU	1 pess	x 1	x 14	14 pessaries
	Helminthic infections					
120.0	Schistosomiasis haematobia					
	Adults	Metrifonate 100 mg	4.5 tabs stat, then			
			repeat after 2 and 4 weeks			13.5 tabs
	Children	Metrifonate 100 mg	1 tab stat, then			
			repeat after 2 and 4 weeks			3 tabs
	NB: Praziquantel may be used as an alternative, in an average dosis as for S. mansoni					
120.1	Schistosomiasis mansoni					
	Adults	Praziquantel 600 mg	4 tabs	stat		4 tabs
	Children	Praziquantel 600 mg	1 1/2 tabs	stat		1 1/2 tabs
120.2	Schistosomiasis japonica					
	Adults	Praziquantel 600 mg	3 tabs	x 2	x 1	6 tabs
	Children	Praziquantel 600 mg	2 tabs	x 1	x 2	4 tabs
123.3	Taeniasis (tapeworm)					
	Adults	Niclosamide 500 mg	4 tabs	stat		4 tabs
	Children	Niclosamide 500 mg	2 tabs	stat		2 tabs
	or: Adults	Praziquantel 600 mg	1 tab	stat		1 tab
	Children	Praziquantel 600 mg	0.25 tab	stat		0.25 tab
125.3	Onchocerciasis (river blindness)					
	Severity 1 (light infections without severe eye complications but only in cases with severe itching and/or dermatitis)					
	Adults	Diethylcarbamazine 50 mg	1 tab	x 1	x 1	
			then 2 tabs	x 1	x 1	
			then 4 tabs	x 1	x 5	23 tabs
	Children	Diethylcarbamazine 50 mg	1/2 tab	x 1	x 1	
			then 1 tab	x 1	x 1	
			then 2 tabs	x 1	x 5	11.5 tabs
	Severity 2 (high risk individuals with heavy ocular microfilarial load):					
	Adults	Suramin sodium 1 gram	wk 1: 0.2 g IV inj			
			wk 2: 0.4 g IV inj			
			wk 3: 0.6 g IV inj			
			wk 4: 0.8 g IV inj			
			wk 5&6: 1 g IV inj			6 vials
	Children	Suramin sodium 1 gram	adapted dose			assume 2 vials
	NB: Treatment with suramin should always be preceeded by treatment with diethylcarbamazine					
	NB: Treatment with suramin sodium only to be given under close medical supervision					

continued

Table 5.1A (continued)

ICD	INDICATION	DRUGS	DOSE	TIMES PER DAY	NO.OF DAYS	AMOUNT PER COURSE OF TREATMENT
125	Other filarial infections					
	Adults	Diethylcarbamazine 50 mg	1/2 tab	x 2	x 1	
			then 1 tab	x 2	x 1	
			then 2 tabs	x 2	x 1	
			then 3 tabs	x 3	x 11	106 tabs
126	Hookworm	Mebendazole 100 mg	1 tab	x 2	x 3	6 tabs
	NB: Many of these patients will have iron deficiency anaemia, which may need additional treatment					
127.0	Ascariasis (roundworm)	Mebendazole 100 mg	1 tab	x 2	x 3	6 tabs
	NB: Pyrantel could be used as an alternative					
	Other parasitic infections					
131.0	Trichomonas, vaginal	Metronidazole 250 mg	8 tabs	stat		8 tabs
132	Pediculosis (lice)	Lindane cream 1%	apply, repeat after one week			1 tube
133.0	Scabies	Benzylbenzoate lotion 25%	apply	x 1	x 2	60 ml
	2. ENDOCRINE, NUTRITIONAL AND METABOLIC DISORDERS					
250	Diabetes Mellitus					
	Severity 1 (non-insulin dependent):					
	Adults	diet				
		Glibenclamide 4 mg	1-3 tabs	x 1	x 28	assume 56 tabs
	Severity 2 (juvenile onset and/or insulin dependent);					
	Adults	Comp Insulin Zinc Susp	20-80 IU (av.60)	x 1	x 28	4.5 vials 400 IU
	Children	Comp Insulin Zinc Susp	10-50 IU (av.30)	x 1	x 28	2.1 vials 400 IU
260-3	Malnutrition					
	Nutritional supplements to be decided locally					
264	Vitamin A deficiency, xerophthalmia					
	Adults & Children >1 y	Vitamin A (retinol) 200000 IU	1 caps stat, repeat after 1 day and 2-4 weeks			3 caps
265-9	Other vitamin deficiency	Food or vitamin supplements to be decided locally.				
	4. DISEASES OF BLOOD AND BLOODFORMING ORGANS					
280	Iron deficiency anaemia					
	Adults	Ferrous sulfate (60 mg iron)	1 tab	x 3	x 28	84 tabs
	Children	Ferrous sulfate (60 mg iron)	1 tab	x 1	x 28	28 tabs
	NB: Iron dextran injection could be substituted in some cases					
282.5	Sickle cell disease					
	Adults	Folic acid 1 mg	5 tabs weekly			20 tabs
	Children 1-5 y	Folic acid 1 mg	2 tabs weekly			8 tabs
	Children <1 y	Folic acid 1 mg	1 tab weekly			4 tabs
	5. MENTAL DISORDERS					
290-9	Psychosis					
	Adults	Chlorpromazine 100 mg	1 tab	x 3	x 7	21 tabs
	Children	Chlorpromazine 100 mg	1/4 tab	x 2	x 7	3.5 tabs
300.0	Anxiety neurosis	Diazepam 5 mg	1 tab	x 3	x 7	21 tabs
300.4	Depressive neurosis	Imipramine 25 mg	1 tab	x 3	x 7	21 tabs
	NB Treatment with antidepressant drugs should be continued for at least one month					

continued

Table 5.1A (continued)

ICD	INDICATION	DRUGS	DOSE	TIMES PER DAY	NO.OF DAYS	AMOUNT PER COURSE OF TREATMENT
	6. DISEASES OF THE NERVOUS SYSTEM AND SENSE ORGANS					
345.0	Petit-mal epilepsy					
	Adults	Phenobarbital 50 mg	1 tab	x 3	x 28	84 tabs
	Children	Phenobarbital 50 mg	5-8 mg/kg/day assume 1/2 tab	x 3	x 28	42 tabs
345.1	Grand-mal epilepsy					
	Adults	Phenobarbital 50 mg	1 tab	x 3	x 28	84 tabs
		or Phenytoin 100 mg	1/2 tab	x 3	x 28	42 tabs
	Children	Phenobarbital 50 mg	5-8 mg/kg/day assume 1/2 tab	x 3	x 28	42 tabs
		or Phenytoin 100 mg	5-8 mg/kg/day assume 1/4 tab	x 3	x 28	21 tabs
345.3	Status epilepticus	Diazepam 10 mg/2 ml	10-20 mg slow IV inj stat			
372.0	Conjunctivitis	Tetracycline eye ointment 1%	apply	x 3	x 7	1 tube 5 g
380.1	Otitis externa					
	Adults	Aluminium acetate 13% drops	3-4 drops	x 4	x 5	10 ml
		Acetylsalicylic acid 300 mg	2 tabs	x 4	x 1	8 tabs
	Children	Aluminium acetate 13% drops	3-4 drops	x 4	x 5	10 ml
		Paracetamol 500 mg	1/2 tab	x 4	x 1	2 tabs
381.2	Otitis media					
	Adults	Sulfameth/trim 400/80 mg	2 tabs	x 2	x 5	20 tabs
		Paracetamol 500 mg	2 tabs	x 4	x 2	16 tabs
	Children	Sulfameth/trim 400/80 mg	1 tab	x 2	x 5	10 tabs
		Paracetamol 500 mg	1/2 tab	x 4	x 2	4 tabs
	7. DISEASES OF THE CIRCULATORY SYSTEM					
390-8	Rheumatic heart disease					
	Adults & Children	Benzath benz penicill 2.4 MU	1.2 MU inj IM	once per month		1/2 vial
	NB: Treatment to be continued till the patient is 18 years of age, or for 5 years if that is longer					
401-5	Hypertension	Saltfree diet				
		Hydrochlorothiazide 50 mg	1-2 tabs	x 1	x 28	56 tabs
410-4	Ischaemic heart disease	Glyceryl trinitrate 0.5 mg	1/2 tab	as required		assume 4 tabs
	NB: Patients with frequent attacks that do not respond to glyceryl trinitrate should be referred.					
455	Haemorrhoids	Hydrocortisone 1% ointment	apply as required			1 tube 15 g
459	Shock	Dextran 70	as required			assume 1 ltr
	8. DISEASES OF THE RESPIRATORY SYSTEM					
460	Common cold, catarrh, sore throat					
	Adults	Paracetamol 500 mg	2 tabs	x 4	x 1	8 tabs
	Children	Supportive measures including fluids and regular review				
		Paracetamol 500 mg	1/2 tab	x 4	x 2	4 tabs
463	Tonsillitis (bacterial, with adenitis)					
	Adults	Procaine benzylpenicillin 3 MU	1 MU inj IM	stat		1/3 vial
		Phenoxymethylpenicillin 250 mg	2 tabs	x 4	x 5	40 tabs
		Paracetamol 500 mg	2 tabs	x 4	x 1	8 tabs
	Children	Phenoxymethylpenicillin 250 mg	1 tab	x 4	x 5	20 tabs
		Paracetamol 500 mg	1/2 tab	x 4	x 2	4 tabs
465	Acute bronchitis					
	Adults	Paracetamol 500 mg	2 tabs	x 4	x 1	8 tabs
	Children	Paracetamol 500 mg	1/2 tab	x 4	x 2	4 tabs
	NB: Most cases of acute bronchitis are viral and of a mild nature; usually no antimicrobials are necessary					

continued

Table 5.1A (continued)

ICD	INDICATION	DRUGS	DOSE	TIMES PER DAY	NO.OF DAYS	AMOUNT PER COURSE OF TREATMENT
480-6	Pneumonia					
	Severity 1 (moderate lower respiratory tract infection with cough, fast breathing but no chest indrawing):					
	Adults	Procaine benzylpenicillin 3 MU	1 MU inj IM	stat		1/3 vial
		Phenoxymethylpenicillin 250 mg	2 tabs	x 4	x 5	40 tabs
		Paracetamol 500 mg	2 tabs	x 4	x 1	8 tabs
	Children	Sulfameth/trim 400/80 mg	1 tab	x 2	x 5	10 tabs
		Paracetamol 500 mg	1/2 tab	x 4	x 2	4 tabs
	Severity 2 (severe lower respiratory tract infection with cough, fast breathing and chest indrawing):					
	Adults	Sulfameth/trim 400/80 mg	2 tabs	x 2	x 5	20 tabs
		Paracetamol 500 mg	2 tabs	x 4	x 1	8 tabs
	Children	Benzyl penicillin 3MU	0.75 MU	x 4	x 5	5 vials
		or: Chloramphenicol 250 mg	1 cap	x 4	x 5	20 caps
		Paracetamol 500 mg	1/2 tab	x 4	x 2	4 tabs
	NB: Chloramphenicol or ampicillin could be substituted as alternatives to sulfameth/trim					
491-2	Chronic bronchitis and emphysema					
	Adults	Tetracycline 250 mg	1 tab	x 4	x 5	20 tabs
		Paracetamol 500 mg	2 tabs	x 4	x 1	8 tabs
493	Asthma					
	Severity 1					
	Adults	Salbutamol 4 mg	1 tab	x 3	x 4	12 tabs
	Children	Salbutamol 4 mg	1/4 tab	x 3	x 4	3 tabs
	Severity 2 (acute asthmatic attack):					
	Adults	Epinephrine 1 mg/ml	0.5 mg slow sc inj stat			1 amp
	Children	Epinephrine 1 mg/ml	0.25 mg slow sc inj stat			1 amp
	9. DISEASES OF THE DIGESTIVE SYSTEM					
521.0	Caries, toothache					
	Adults	Acetylsalicylic acid 300 mg	2 tabs	x 4	x 2	16 tabs
	Children	Paracetamol 500 mg	1/2 tab	x 4	x 2	4 tabs
522.5	Dental abscess					
	Adults	Phenoxymethylpenicillin 250 mg	1 tab	x 4	x 5	20 tabs
		Acetylsalicylic acid 300 mg	2 tabs	x 4	x 2	16 tabs
	Children	Phenoxymethylpenicill 250 mg	1/2 tab	x 4	x 5	10 tabs
		Paracetamol 500 mg	1/2 tab	x 4	x 2	4 tabs
528	Mouth sores	Gentian violet paint	apply	x 3	x 5	assume 10 ml
535-6	Gastritis, heartburn, indigestion					
	Adults	Aluminium hydroxyde 500 mg	2 tabs	x 4	x 3	24 tabs
564.0	Constipation					
	Adults	Senna 7.5 mg	2 tabs	stat		2 tabs
	Children	Senna 7.5 mg	1/2 tab	stat		1/2 tab
	10. DISEASES OF THE GENITO-URINARY SYSTEM					
595	Cystitis					
	Severity 1 (isolated episode in adults):					
	Adults	Sulfameth/trim 400/80 mg	4 tabs	stat		4 tabs
		Paracetamol 500 mg	2 tabs	x 4	x 2	16 tabs
	Severity 2 (recurrent or non-responsive episodes in adults; all episodes in children)					
	Adults	Sulfameth/trim 400/80 mg	2 tabs	x 2	x 10	40 tabs
		Paracetamol 500 mg	2 tabs	x 4	x 2	16 tabs
	Children	Sulfameth/trim 400/80 mg	1 tab	x 2	x 5	10 tabs
		Paracetamol 500 mg	1/2 tab	x 4	x 2	4 tabs
	NB: Ampicillin or nitrofurantoin could be substituted for sulfameth/trim in Severity 2.					
614	Pelvic inflammatory disease					
	Adults	Procaine benzylpenicillin 3 MU	4.5 MU inj IM stat			1.5 vials
		Probenicid 500 mg	2 tabs stat			2 tabs
		Tetracycline 250 mg	1 tab	x 4	x 5	20 tabs
		Metronidazole 250 mg	2 tabs	x 3	x 5	30 tabs

continued

Table 5.1A (continued)

ICD	INDICATION		DRUGS	DOSE	TIMES PER DAY	NO.OF DAYS	AMOUNT PER COURSE OF TREATMENT
	11. COMPLICATIONS OF PREGNANCY, CHILDBIRTH AND PUERPERIUM						
634-8	Abortion		Ergometrine 0.2 mg/ml	0.2 mg IM inj (may be repeated)			assume 2 amp
			Ergometrine 0.2 mg	1 tab	x 3	x 3	9 tabs
650	Normal delivery		Ergometrine 0.2 mg/ml	0.2 mg IM inj	stat		1 amp
660-5	Abnormal delivery		Ergometrine 0.2 mg/ml	0.5 mg IM inj	stat		2.5 amp
		NB: For abnormal delivery referral to a hospital will usually be necessary					
666	Postpartum bleeding		Ergometrine 0.2 mg/ml	0.5 mg IM inj (repeat, if necessary)	stat		assume 5 amp
			Dextran 70 infusion	as required			assume 1 ltr
670	Major puerperal infection		Ampicillin 250 mg	2 caps	x 4	x 5	40 caps
675	Mastitis, breast abscess		Procaine benzylpenicillin 3 MU	1 MU inj IM	stat		1/3 vial
			Phenoxymethylpenicillin 250 mg	2 tabs	x 4	x 2	16 tabs
			Paracetamol 500 mg	2 tabs	x 4	x 1	8 tabs
	12. DISEASES OF THE SKIN AND SUBCUTANEOUS TISSUE						
680-2	Boil, abscess						
		Adults	Procaine benzylpenicillin 3 MU	1 MU inj IM	stat		1/3 vial
			Phenoxymethylpenicillin 250 mg	2 tabs	x 4	x 5	40 tabs
			Paracetamol 500 mg	2 tabs	x 4	x 1	8 tabs
		Children	Procaine benzylpenicillin 3 MU	0.3 MU inj IM	stat		1/10 vial
			Phenoxymethylpenicill 250 mg	1/2 tab	x 4	x 5	10 tabs
			Paracetamol 500 mg	1/2 tab	x 4	x 1	2 tabs
		NB: In some cases surgical opening of the abcess and/or disinfection of the skin may be necessary					
684	Bacterial skin infection		Neomycin & Bacitracin ointment	apply	x 4	x 5	1 tube 20 g
691.8	Eczema		Hydrocortisone ointment 1%	apply	x 3	x 7	1 tube 15 g
692	Skin allergy						
		Adults	Chlorphenamine 4 mg	1 tab	x 3	x 4	12 tabs
		Children	Chlorphenamine 4 mg	1/2 tab	x 3	x 4	6 tabs
698	Itching		Calamine lotion	as required			assume 50 ml
707.9	Chronic/tropical ulcer						
		Adults	Procaine benzylpenicillin 3 MU	1 MU inj IM	stat		1/3 vial
			Phenoxymethylpenicillin 250 mg	2 tabs	x 4	x 5	40 tabs
			Gentian violet paint	apply	x 3	x 5	assume 10 ml
	13. DISEASES OF THE MUSCULOSKELETAL SYSTEM AND CONNECTIVE TISSUE						
714-6	Arthritis and arthrosis						
		Adults	Acetylsalicylic acid 300 mg	2 tabs	x 4	x 5	40 tabs
724	Backpain, lumbago						
		Adults	Acetylsalicylic acid 300 mg	2 tabs	x 4	x 5	40 tabs
728	Pyomyositis						
		Adults	Chloramphenicol 1 gram	1 g IM inj	stat		1 vial
			Chloramphenicol 250 mg	2 caps	x 4	x 7	56 caps
			Acetylsalicylic acid 300 mg	2 tabs	x 4	x 2	16 caps
		Children	Chloramphenicol 1 gram	0.25 g IM inj	stat		1/4 vial
			Chloramphenicol 250 mg	1 caps	x 3	x 7	21 caps
			Paracetamol 500 mg	1/2 tab	x 4	x 2	4 tabs
	16. SYMPTOMS, SIGNS AND ILL-DEFINED CONDITIONS						
780.3	Convulsions, febrile						
		Adults	Diazepam 10 mg/2 ml	10-20 mg IV inj	stat		assume 2 amp
		Children	Diazepam 10 mg/2 ml	5-10 mg IV inj	stat		assume 1 amp

continued

Table 5.1A (continued)

ICD	INDICATION		DRUGS	DOSE	TIMES PER DAY	NO.OF DAYS	AMOUNT PER COURSE OF TREATMENT
780.5	Insomnia						
		Adults	Diazepam 5 mg	1 tab	x 1	x 14	14 tabs
780.6	Fever NEC						
		Adults	Paracetamol 500 mg	2 tabs	x 4	x 1	8 tabs
		Children	Paracetamol 500 mg	1/2 tab	x 4	x 1	2 tabs
780.7	Malaise, fatigue						
		NB: Local decisions to be taken on whether drugs are to be provided for this group of symptoms					
784.0	Headache						
		Adults	Acetylsalicylic acid 300 mg	2 tabs	x 4	x 1	8 tabs
		Children	Paracetamol 500 mg	1/2 tab	x 4	x 1	2 tabs
786.2	Cough NEC						
		Adults	Chlorphenamine 4 mg	1 tab	x 3	x 2	6 tabs
		Children	Chlorphenamine 4 mg	1/2 tab	x 3	x 2	3 tabs
			or: Promethazine syrup 5 mg/5 ml	5 ml	x 3	x 2	30 ml
787.0	Vomiting						
		Adults	Promethazine 25 mg	1 tab	x 3	x 2	6 tabs
		Children	Promethazine syrup 5 mg/5 ml	5 ml	x 3	x 2	30 ml
788.0	Renal colic						
		Adults	Pethidine 100 mg/2 ml	100 mg IM inj	stat		1 amp
789.0	Abdominal pain NEC						
		Adults	Acetylsalicylic acid 300 mg	2 tabs	x 4	x 1	8 tabs
		Children	Paracetamol 500 mg	1/2 tab	x 4	x 1	2 tabs
	17. INJURY AND POISONING						
800-29	Fractures						
		Adults	Acetylsalicylic acid 300 mg	2 tabs	x 4	x 2	16 tabs
		Children	Paracetamol 500 mg	1/2 tab	x 4	x 2	4 tabs
		NB: Other treatment and/or referral for further treatment will usually be necessary					
830-9	Dislocations						
		Adults	Acetylsalicylic acid 300 mg	2 tabs	x 4	x 1	8 tabs
		Children	Paracetamol 500 mg	1/2 tab	x 4	x 1	2 tabs
		NB: Other treatment and/or referral for further treatment will usually be necessary					
840-8	Sprains and strains						
		Adults	Acetylsalicylic acid 300 mg	2 tabs	x 4	x 1	8 tabs
		Children	Paracetamol 500 mg	1/2 tab	x 4	x 1	2 tabs
850-4	Intracranial injury, concussion						
		Adults	Acetylsalicylic acid 300 mg	2 tabs	x 4	x 2	16 tabs
		Children	Paracetamol 500 mg	1/2 tab	x 4	x 2	4 tabs
		NB: Other supportive measures or referral will usually be necessary					
870-90	Open wound, laceration, major cut						
		Adults	Chlorhexidine conc sol 5%	diluted as required			assume 1 ml
			Lidocaine 1% 50 ml	as required			assume 10 ml
			Acetylsalicylic acid 300 mg	2 tabs	x 4	x 2	16 tabs
		Children	Chlorhexidine conc sol 5%	diluted as required			assume 1 ml
			Lidocaine 1% 50 ml	as required			assume 5 ml
			Paracetamol 500 mg	1/2 tab	x 4	x 2	4 tabs
		NB: Allowance should be made for tetanus toxoid to be given to patients with wounds					
879.9	Complicated open wound, animal or human bite						
		Adults	Chlorhexidine conc sol 5%	diluted as required			assume 1 ml
			Procaine benzylpenicillin 3 MU	1 MU inj IM	stat		1/3 vial
			Phenoxymethylpenicillin 250 mg	2 tabs	x 4	x 5	40 tabs
			Acetylsalicylic acid 300 mg	2 tabs	x 4	x 1	8 tabs
		Children	Chlorhexidine conc sol 5%	diluted as required			assume 1 ml
			Procaine benzylpenicillin 3 MU	0.3 MU inj IM	stat		1/10 vial
			Phenoxymethylpenicillin 250 mg	1/2 tab	x 4	x 5	10 tabs
			Paracetamol 500 mg	1/2 tab	x 4	x 1	2 tabs
		NB: Allowance should be made for tetanus toxoid to be given to patients with animal bites					

continued

Table 5.1A (continued)

ICD	INDICATION	DRUGS	DOSE	TIMES PER DAY	NO.OF DAYS	AMOUNT PER COURSE OF TREATMENT
910-19	Superficial injury, bruise, minor cut					
	Adults and children	Chlorhexidine conc sol 5%	diluted as required			assume 1 ml
	NB: Allowance should be made for tetanus toxoid to be given to patients with wounds					
930	Foreign body in eye					
	for diagnosis:	Fluoresceine eye drops 1%	apply a one drop in the eye			
	for treatment:	Tetracycline eye ointment 1%	apply	x 3	x 2	1 tube 5 g
940-9	Burns, all degrees					
	Adults	Chlorhexidine conc sol 5%	diluted as required			assume 1 ml
		Acetylsalicylic acid 300 mg	2 tabs	x 4	x 1	8 tabs
	Children	Chlorhexidine conc sol 5%	diluted as required			assume 1 ml
		Paracetamol 500 mg	1/2 tab	x 4	x 1	2 tabs
960-79	Poisoning					
	Adults	Ipacacuanha 0.14% syrup	30 ml stat			30 ml
	Children	Ipacacuanha 0.14% syrup	15 ml stat			15 ml
989.5	Snake bite, other stings and bites					
	Snake bite	Antivenom sera	30-100 ml slow IV inj			assume 50 ml
	NB: Referral to a specialist center may be necessary					
	Insect bites and stings					
	Adults	Chlorhexidine conc sol 5%	diluted as required			assume 1 ml
		Chlorphenamine 4 mg	1 tab	x4	x 2	8 tabs
	Children	Chlorhexidine conc sol 5%	diluted as required			assume 1 ml
		Chlorphenamine 4 mg	1/2 tab	x 3	x 2	3 tabs
995.0	Anaphylactic shock					
	Adults	Epinephrine 1 mg/ml	0.5 mg slow sc inj			assume 1 amp
	Children	Epinephrine 1 mg/ml	0.25 mg slow sc inj			assume 1 amp
	NB: This treatment may be repeated, if necessary					
	OTHER HEALTH SERVICE CONTACTS					
V03-06	Vaccinations	See Expanded Programme of Immunization (EPI)				
V20	Under-five preventive care	Drug treatment, if necessary, to be decided locally				
V22-23.	Antenatal care	Ferrous sulphate 60 mg iron with Folic acid 0.25 mg	1 tab	x 2	x 28	56 tabs per month
V25	Family planning, contraception	See Family Planning Programme				
V70	Medical Examination, no disease	Placebo treatment, if necessary, to be decided locally				

KEY

benzath benzylpenicill	benzathine benzylpenicillin
caps	capsule(s)
conc	concentrate
INH	isoniazid
ointm	ointment
oral rehydr salts	oral rehydration salts, ORS
sol	solution
stat	statim, immediately
sulfameht/trim	sulfamethoxazole and trimethoprim
susp	suspension

Table 5.1B
Alphabetical list of diseases and complaints for the middle level

(numbers refer to ICD classification in main table)

Disease/complaint	ICD	Disease/complaint	ICD	Disease/complaint	ICD
Abscess	680-2	Dislocations	830-9	Pelvic inflammatory disease	614
Abdominal pain	789.0	Eczema	691.8	Pneumonia	480-6
Abortion	634-8	Emphysema	491-2	Poisoning	960-79
Amoebiasis	006-7	Epilepsy, grand mal	345.1	Postpartum bleeding	666
Anaemia	280	Epilepsy, petit mal	345.0	Psychosis	290-9
Anaphylactic shock	995.0	Epilepsy, status	345.3	Puerperal infection, major	670
Ancylostomiasis	126	Eye, foreign body in	930	Pyomyositis	728
Antenatal care	V22-23	Family planning	V25	Renal colic	788.0
Anticonception	V25	Fatigue	780.7	Rheumatic heart disease	390-8
Anxiety neurosis	300.0	Fever	780.6	River blindness	125.3
Arthritis	714-6	Filaria, other	125	Roundworm	127.0
Arthrosis	714-6	Foreign body in eye	930	Scabies	133.0
Ascariasis	127.0	Fractures	800-29	Schistosomiasis haematobia	120.0
Asthma	493	Gastritis	535-6	Schistosomiasis japonica	120.2
Bacillary dysentery	004	Gastroenteritis	009.2	Schistosomiasis mansoni	120.1
Backpain	724	Giardiasis	006-7	Shock, anaphylactic	995.0
Bite, animal	879.9	Gonorrhoea	098.0	Shock, hypovolaemic459	
Bite, human	879.9	Haemorrhoids	455	Sickle cell disease	282.5
Bite, other	989.5	Headache	784.0	Skin allergy	692
Bite, snake	989.5	Heartburn	535-6	Skin infection, bacterial	684
Boil	680-2	Hookworm	126	Skin infection, fungal	110
Breast abscess	675	Hypertension	401-5	Snake bite	989.5
Bronchitis, acute	465	Indigestion	535.6	Sore throat	460
Bronchitis, chronic	491-2	Injury, superficial	910-19	Sprains and strains	840-8
Bruise	910-19	Insomnia	780.5	Status epilepticus	345.3
Burns, all degrees	940-9	Intracranial injury	850-4	Stings, insect	989.5
Candidiasis, vaginal	112.1	Iron deficiency anaemia	280	Syphilis	090-7
Caries	521.0	Ischaemic heart disease	410-4	Taeniasis	123.3
Catarrh	460	Itching	698	Tapeworm	123.3
Chickenpox	052	Laceration	870-90	Tonsillitis, bacterial	463
Cholera	001	Leprosy	030	Toothache	521.0
Common cold	460	Lice	132	Trachoma	076
Concussion	850-4	Lumbago	724	Trichomonas, vaginal	131.0
Conjunctivitis	372.0	Malaise	780.7	Tropical ulcer	707.9
Constipation	564.0	Malaria	084	Tuberculosis, pulmonary	011
Contraception	V25	Malnutrition	260-3	Typhoid	002.0
Convulsions, febrile	780.3	Mastitis	675	Ulcer, chronic	707.9
Cough	786.2	Measles	055	Ulcer, tropical	707.9
Cutwound, major	870-90	Medical Examination	V70	Under-five preventive care	V20
Cutwound, minor	910-19	Mouth sores	528	Vaccinations	V03-06
Cystitis	595	Onchocerciasis	125.3	Vitamin A deficiency	264
Delivery, abnormal	660-5	Open wound, complicated	879.9	Vitamin deficiency, other	265-9
Delivery, normal	650	Open wound, simple	870-90	Vomiting	787.0
Dental abscess	522.5	Ophthalmia neonatorum	098.4	Xerophthalmia	264
Depressive neurosis	300.4	Otitis externa	380.1		
Diabetes Mellitus	250	Otitis media	381.2		
Diarrhoea, acute	009.2	Pediculosis	132		

Publications relevant to drug treatment therapy

Gross F, et al. (1984). Management of Arterial Hypertension. A Practical Guide for the Physician and Allied Health Workers. Geneva: WHO.

Federal Ministry of Health, Nigeria (1980). National Basic Health Services Scheme: Standing Orders. Lagos: Federal Ministry of Health.

Joint Formulary Committee (1987). British National Formulary, Number 14. London: British Medical Association and the Pharmaceutical Society of Great Britain.

Manson-Bahr PEC, Apted FIC Eds. (1982). Manson's Tropical Diseases, 18th Edition. London: Balliere Tindall.

Ministry of Health, Sri Lanka (1987). Manual on Management of Drugs. Colombo: Ministry of Health, Government of the Democratic Socialistic Republic of Sri Lanka.

Ministry of Health, Zimbabwe (1985). EDLIZ Essential Drug List for Zimbabwe, including Guidelines for Treatment of Medical Conditions in Zimbabwe. Harare: Ministry of Health.

Petit P (1979). Management Schedules for Dispensaries. Nairobi: African Medical and Research Foundation.

Schull CR (1980). Standard Management of Common Medical Problems of Adults in Papua New Guinea. Madang: Kristen Press Inc.

Upanda G, et al. (1983). Guideline to Drug Usage. London: Macmillan Press.

WHO (1982). Control of Vitamin A Deficiency and Xerophthalmia. Technial Report Series 672. Geneva: WHO.

WHO (1983). The Role of Chemotherapy in Schistosomiasis Control. WHO/SCHISTO/83.70 Rev 1. Geneva: WHO.

WHO (1984a). Malaria Control as Part of Primary Health Care. Technical Report Series 712. Geneva: WHO.

WHO (1984b). Advances in Malaria Chemotherapy. Technical Report Series 711. Geneva: WHO.

WHO (1984c). A Manual for the Treatment of Acute Diarrhoea. For Use by Physicians and other Senior Health Workers. WHO/CDD/SER/80.2 REV 1. Geneva: WHO.

WHO (1984d). Strategies for the Prevention of Blindness in National Programmes - Primary Health Care Approach. Geneva: WHO.

WHO (1985a). Case Management of Acute Respiratory Infections in Children in Developing Countries. WHO/RSD/85.15 Rev 2. Geneva: WHO.

WHO (1985b). Diabetes Mellitus. Technical Report Series 722. Geneva: WHO.

WHO (1985c). Simplified Approaches for Sexually Transmitted Disease (STD) Control at the Primary Health Care (PHC) Level. WHO/VDT/85.437. Geneva: WHO.

WHO (1986a). Respiratory Infections in Children: Management at Small Hospitals. Background Notes and a Manual for Doctors. WHO/RSD/86.26. Geneva: WHO.

WHO (1986b). WHO Expert Committee on Venereal Diseases and Treponematoses. Technical Report Series 736. Geneva: WHO.

WHO, Eastern Mediterranean Region (1985). Rational Use of Essential Drugs in Primary Health Care by the Doctor. WHO/EM/PHARM/102. Alexandria: WHO Regional office for the Eastern Mediterranean.

WHO, Regional Office for the Eastern Mediterranean (1986). Eastern Mediterranean Drug Information Sheets. Drugs for Use at the Primary Health Care Level by Doctors and Community Health Workers. WHO-EM/PHARM/115-E. Alexandria: WHO Regional office for the Eastern Mediterranean.

MODULE 6:

DATA REQUIREMENT: MORBIDITY DATA

1. THE DATA REQUIRED - TREATMENT EPISODES

This module deals with the final data input needed for this method: patient morbidity data.

As explained in Module 1, the basic formula for the morbidity method of quantification is:

Quantity of the drug specified for a standard course of treatment	x	Number of treatment episodes of the health problem	=	Total quantity of a drug required for a given health problem

What we need to know therefore is the number of treatment episodes of each health problem (and of the different standard treatments, if they are different by age group and severity) in the type(s) of health facilities whose drug requirements are being quantified.

Before going on to discuss how such data may be obtained, it will be useful to have a more precise definition of a treatment episode and its relationship to certain other terms such as "total cases", "new cases" and "old cases", which are frequently used in recording health service statistics.

A treatment episode is a patient contact for which a standard course of drug treatment is required.

Four points in this definition merit further explanation:

(a) What distinguishes a treatment episode from other contacts is that **it requires a standard drug treatment.**

If a standard treatment is specified for a particular health problem, then a new patient contact for this problem counts as a treatment episode. However, if this patient has to return for repeat contacts before the problem is cured, each repeat visit, where the standard treatment is again required, also counts as a treatment episode. If no new drug treatment is required, for example because the repeat visit is for a follow-up check on the patient's progress, then it does not count as a treatment episode.

EXAMPLE:

A patient contacts a health centre, and anaemia is diagnosed. A first standard drug treatment is given. This contact is recorded as a new contact - or a new case of anaemia, and it is the first treatment episode. The patient is then told to return for a check-up. If at this next visit another course of treatment is given, this visit counts as a treatment episode. After the drugs have been stopped, the patient may again be asked to return for one or more check-ups to be sure that he or she is cured. Since no drug treatment is required at these check-up visits they do not count as treatment episodes.

(b) A single **patient contact** may give rise to more than one treatment episode, if several health problems are diagnosed and a standard course of drug treatment is required for each one.

EXAMPLE:

Suppose that the case diagnosed as anaemia returns as instructed for a repeat prescription of the standard treatment, and is found to have two other health problems, for example, a worm infestation and an upper respiratory tract infection, and that a standard treatment is also required for each of these problems. This contact will have given rise to three treatment episodes, one for each health problem.

(c) The definition of a treatment episode uses the phrase "for which a standard course of drug treatment is **required**". There are at least two reasons for this:

If drugs are in short supply, it may not be possible to give the standard treatment required. What we need to know then is the number of standard courses of treatment **required** for each health problem, not those actually given. If, on the other hand, a patient returns for a check-up and no further drug treatment is prescribed, the visit does not count as a new treatment episode.

(d) What we need to know **is the number of treatment episodes** for which a standard treatment was prescribed. Where a particular health problem has several different standard treatments for different age groups or severities, then the number of treatment episodes for **each** of these must be established separately.

EXAMPLE:

Turn back to Table 5.1. For health problem 132, Pediculosis (lice), there is only one average standard drug treatment, and only the total number of treatment episodes is required.

In contrast, for health problem 084, Malaria, four different average treatments are specified depending on whether the patient is a child or an adult, and whether the problem is mild or severe. The number of treatment episodes for each of the four average treatments is required.

2. TASK 11: DATA COLLECTION

There are three options for collecting the necessary data on the numbers of treatment episodes of each standard treatment:

(1) to use **centrally assembled patient morbidity data** if these are available;

(2) to **estimate** the numbers from **routine patient records** at a **sample** of health facilities;

(3) or, if this is not possible, to **collect** the necessary statistics **prospectively** from a **sample** of health facilities.

Whichever of those methods is used, it must be emphasized in the strongest possible terms that **the quality of the final estimate of drugs required will only be as good as the quality of the morbidity data. If the morbidity data are seriously incomplete or unreliable, then the drug estimate may be dangerously inadequate or inappropriate.**

2.1 Estimates from centrally assembled patient morbidity data

In most countries health facilities keep patient records of one kind or another, such as day books, registers, or record cards, in which details of patients attending for care are recorded. These records usually contain some or all of the following items for each contact:

a) date of contact/admission/discharge,
b) diagnosis or purpose of contact (and possibly whether the contact is a new one or a repeat),
c) age or age group,

d) sex,
e) treatment given,
f) patient's name (at least for patients admitted for in-patient care).

In some countries these data are assembled at regional and national level, for epidemiological and planning purposes. There is a considerable saving of time and effort if these data can be used for estimating the number of treatment episodes of each health problem. The four main steps for making this estimate are listed in Table 6.1 and briefly explained below.

Table 6.1
Estimating treatment episodes from national level patient morbidity statistics

STEP 1:	Obtain the total numbers of patient contacts by diagnosis in the type(s) of health facilities whose drug needs are to be quantified.
STEP 2:	Reorganize the diagnoses according to the health problems defined in the average standard treatments.
STEP 3:	Within health problems, break down the number of patient contacts as necessary by age group and severity.
STEP 4:	Determine the proportion of contacts for which a standard treatment is required.

STEP 1: Obtain the total numbers of patient contacts by diagnosis in the type(s) of health facilities whose drug needs are to be quantified.

These data will be aggregated statistics from the statistical reports sent in by individual facilities, to the central statistics or health information unit. **It is absolutely crucial that these statistics be complete.** If they are not complete, for example because the health facilities concerned tend to under-record, or because some have not sent in their statistics, then the drug estimates will also be incomplete. The extent of any incompleteness must be evaluated and corrected. For example, if certain health facilities have not sent in their statistics, they must either be asked to do so immediately, or their numbers of patient contacts must be estimated and added to the national total.

It is also crucial that these statistics be reliable. Errors arising from poor record keeping, such as filling in diagnoses from memory every few days, will be directly reflected in the drug estimates.

STEP 2: Reorganize the diagnoses according to the health problems defined in the average standard treatments.

As already explained in Module 5, a health problem may include several diagnoses with the same average standard treatment. The basic statistics by diagnosis need therefore to be grouped and reorganized to match the list of health problems for which average standard treatments have been specified. For example, in the illustrative average standard treatment schedules shown in Table 5.1, the health problem "lower respiratory tract infection" includes all ICD diagnoses from 480 to 486.

These groupings can be done only **if the diagnoses recorded are sufficiently detailed.** For example, in Table 5.1, under diseases of the respiratory system, six different health problems are distinguished. If the diagnostic data in the routine statistics simply grouped all respiratory diseases, there would be no reliable way of breaking down the total number of patient contacts among the five health problems specified.

STEP 3: Within health problems, break down the number of patient contacts as necessary by age group and severity.

Where different average standard treatments are specified within a health problem, according to the patient's age group, (child/adult), or the severity of the disease (mild/severe) or both, the number of patient contacts for **each one** must be established. For example, in Module 5, Table 5.1, we saw that four average standard treatments were specified within the health problem malaria. It is necessary to establish the number of patient contacts for all four.

(a) Contacts by age group

If a country has developed its patient morbidity statistics to the point of assembling them nationally, it is quite likely that they will distinguish between children and adults. If this distinction is not made, then there are three possible options: estimate from experience, demographic statistics, or do a sample survey.

The quickest method is to ask experienced clinicians to estimate the relative proportions of child and adult contacts, for each health problem where different standard treatments are specified for children and adults. But the answer will be rough, and the likely margin of error may cause the estimated drug requirement to be 10-20% above or below the real requirement.

EXAMPLE:

Suppose that for a particular health problem, children require 5 tablets for an average standard treatment and adults require twice this, that is 10 tablets (this ratio of 2:1 is quite common - see Table 5.I). If, in every 1,000 contacts for this health problem, 200 are adults and 800 are children, and all require a standard treatment, the drug requirement per 1,000 contacts is 6,000 tablets (200 x 10) + (800 x 5). However, if the clinicians estimate that 400 are adults and 600 are children, the estimated drug requirement would be 7,000 tablets (400 x 10) + (600 x 5) or almost 17% above the real requirement.

Alternatively, suppose the real proportions are the other way around, that is, 800 adults and 200 children, the total drug requirement per 1,000 contacts is 9,000 tablets (800 x 10) + (200 x 5). If the clinicians estimate 600 adults and 400 children, the estimated drug requirement will be 8,000 tablets (600 x 10) + (400 x 5) or over 11% below the real requirement.

The alternative is to do a sample survey of the type(s) of facilities concerned. It may be that though data are not tabulated by age, it is actually noted in patient records. If this is so then a retrospective review of patient records from a sample of health facilities can be done relatively quickly to determine the proportions of adults and children.

If no age data are recorded, then a prospective survey must be done to record these data, and this will take considerably longer.

(b) Contacts by severity

It is highly unlikely that national patient morbidity data will distinguish different levels of severity within diagnoses. The quickest, but again the roughest way to establish this breakdown is once more to estimate from clinical experience. For example, it might be estimated that of all health centre contacts for malaria, 60% are adults and 40% are children, and that 10% of the children and 5% of the adults are severe cases. Evidently, if clinical estimates are used for both age group and severity, the potential margin of error is increased.

The alternative is to do a sample survey of the type(s) of facilities concerned. If the patient records are detailed enough then a retrospective review can be done. For example, diagnostic data may be accompanied by clinical notes indicating severity, such as: malaria - with severe fever; acute diarrhoea - with over 10% dehydration; onchocerciasis - with heavy ocular load of microfilaria. In the absence of such notes, treatment information may be recorded, which allow severity to be deduced. For example: malaria - quinine injections; measles - procaine benzylpenicillin injections; onchocerciasis - suramin sodium injections, leave no doubt that these are severe cases.

If records do not indicate severity or allow it to be deduced, then a prospective sample survey must be done.

STEP 4: Determine the proportion of contacts for which a standard treatment is required.

Once steps 1-3 above have been completed, we have the estimated number of patient contacts for each standard drug treatment. As discussed in section 1 above, a standard treatment is not necessarily given or required at every contact. We must therefore determine the proportion of contacts who require a standard treatment.

The simplest method is to estimate the proportion of contacts requiring a standard treatment on the basis of staff experience. As already explained above, such estimates can involve a significant margin of error.

The alternative is again a sample survey - based on retrospective data if the patient records are good enough, or if not then a prospective survey. Table 6.2 shows a typical work-sheet for recording these calculations.

One further point must be borne in mind. Whatever method of data collection is used, the results will be the number of treatment episodes **in the past,** whereas we wish to quantify drug requirements for **future** orders. If it is known that the use of the health services we are dealing with is increasing or falling, then the estimates of the number of treatment episodes should be adjusted up or down to allow for the expected changes.

EXAMPLE:

Suppose that health service use is increasing at 3% annually because of population growth. If the latest morbidity data are two years old and we are estimating next year's requirements, then for every 1,000 treatment episodes two years ago we may expect 1,092 next year (1,000 x 1.03 x 1.03 x 1.03).

2.2 Estimate from morbidity data from a sample of health facilities

Many developing countries record fairly detailed patient morbidity data at the operational level in individual health facilities, but do not assemble these data centrally. In such cases, the calculations described above for national data may be done on patient morbidity data from a representative sample of health facilities. The size of the sample, and the choice of representative facilities involve technical issues beyond the scope of this manual and should be decided in collaboration with statisticians and epidemiologists.

The result of such an estimate would be one worksheet, similar to Table 6.2, giving the number of treatment episodes for each health facility in the sample. These worksheets then have to be consolidated to obtain the total sample results. Table 6.3 shows a typical consolidation worksheet for adding the results from each facility.

This calculation gives only the number of treatment episodes of each standard treatment for the facilities in the sample. These numbers therefore need to be scaled up to obtain the national figures. In order to calculate the scaling up factor we first need to know the total number of contacts at all the facilities of the type(s) included in the quantification.

Table 6.2
Work sheet for calculating treatment episodes

Name......................... Location...

1 ICD Code	2 Health problem	3 Number of contacts Children	4 Adults	5 Total	6 Number of treatment episodes Children	7 Adults	8 Total
009.2	Acute diarrhoea:						
	Severity 1						
	Severity 2						
	Malaria (severity 1)						
084	Ascariasis (roundworm)						
127.0	Pediculosis (lice)						
132	Scabies						
133.0	Iron deficiency anaemia						
280	Conjunctivitis						
372.0	Common cold						
460	Caries, toothache						
521.0	Gastritis,heartburn,indigestion						
535-6	Constipation						
564.0	Cystitis:						
595	Severity 1						
	Severity 2						
	Boil, abscess						
680-2	Impetigo,bacterial skin infection						
684	Chronic arthritis and arthrosis						
714-6	Back-pain, lumbago						
724	Fever NEC						
780.6	Malaise, fatigue NEC						
780.7	Headache NEC						
784.0	Cough NEC						
786.2	Abdominal pain NEC						
789.0	Sprains and strains						
840-8	Superficial injury,bruise,cut						
910-19	Burns						
940-9							
TOTAL							
OTHER HEALTH SERVICE CONTACTS							
V03-06	Vaccinations						
	Under-five preventive care						
V20-							
	Antenatal care						
V22-3							
	Family planning,contraception						
V25							
	Medical examination, no disease						
V70							
TOTAL							

Table 6.3
Consolidation worksheet for number of treatment episodes at all sample facilities

ICD Code	Health problem	Facility 1 Children	Facility 1 Adults	Facility 1 Total	Facility 2 Children	Facility 2 Adults	Facility 2 Total	Facility 3 etc Children	Facility 3 etc Adults	Facility 3 etc Total
009.2	Acute diarrhoea:									
	Severity 2									
	Severity 3									
084	Malaria (severity 1)									
127.0	Ascariasis (roundworm)									
132	Pediculosis (lice)									
133.0	Scabies									
280	Iron deficiency anaemia									
372.0	Conjunctivitis									
460	Common cold									
521.0	Caries, toothache									
535-6	Gastritis,heartburn,indigestion									
564.0	Constipation									
595	Cystitis									
	Severity 1									
	Severity 2									
680-2	Boil, abscess									
684	Impetigo,bacterial skin infection									
714-6	Chronic arthritis and arthrosis									
724	Back-pain, lumbago									
780.6	Fever NEC									
780.7	Malaise, fatigue NEC									
784.0	Headache NEC									
786.2	Cough NEC									
789.0	Abdominal pain NEC									
840-8	Sprains and strains									
910-19	Superficial injury,bruise,cut									
940-9	Burns									
TOTAL										
OTHER HEALTH SERVICE CONTACTS										
V03-06	Vaccinations									
V20	Under-five preventive care									
V22-3	Antenatal care									
V25	Family planning,contraception									
V70	Medical examination, no disease									
TOTAL										

$$\text{The scaling up factor} = \frac{\text{Total patient contacts at all facilities covered by the quantification}}{\text{Total patient contacts at the facilities in the sample}}$$

Then:

Overall total number of treatment episodes for the standard treatment concerned	=	Total number of treatment episodes of that standard treatment at the sample facilities	x	Scaling up factor

EXAMPLE:

Suppose that we are estimating drug requirements for health centres. It is known that they have a total of 10,000,000 patient contacts annually. Patient morbidity records are kept, but not collated centrally. We therefore do a survey of patient records at a sample of health centres. Our survey shows that these health centres have 50,000 patient contacts of which 45,000 are treatment episodes (that is contacts where a standard treatment was given or required) the remainder being repeat visits and visits for preventive services without a standard treatment. For simplicity, suppose there are only five health problems A-E, each with a standard treatment, and that the number of treatment episodes for each are as shown in column 2 of the table below.

The scaling up factor (total contacts/sample contacts) = 10,000,000/50,000 = 200. Multiplying the sample numbers by the scaling up factor, in this case 200, gives the total number of treatment episodes nationally, as shown in column 4 of the table below.

Standard treatment	*Number of treatment episodes in sample facilities*	X	*Scaling up factor*	=	*National total number of treatment episodes*
A	*5,000*		*200*		*1,000,000*
B	*10,000*		"		*2,000,000*
C	*20,000*		"		*4,000,000*
D	*2,500*		"		*500,000*
E	*7,500*		"		*1,500,000*
Total	*45,000*				*9,000,000*

2.3 Prospective sample survey

If the morbidity data available do not record age group and severity, and do not distinguish contacts with standard treatments from contacts for other reasons, a series of estimates have to be made. These estimates can be made quickly on the basis of clinical experience but the margin of error is difficult to judge, and may be relatively large. On the other hand, sample surveys to obtain the missing data can involve almost as much effort as a full scale prospective sample survey.

Therefore, unless existing morbidity data are complete, reliable and detailed, it is usually better to collect the required patient morbidity statistics prospectively. Then they can be tailored precisely to meet the requirements of the calculation so avoiding the various estimates virtually always needed when existing morbidity data are used.

The staff at the sample facilities are briefed to record the number of treatment episodes for each standard treatment on a special record form during several sampling periods throughout the year, to cover the different seasons.

A well designed, easy to use record form is essential to ensure complete and accurate record keeping. An **illustrative example** of such a form is given in Table 6.4. Down the left hand side are listed all the health problems to be treated at this level of care, including all the sub-groups for which a specific standard treatment is indicated in the standard treatment schedules. The health problems used in this illustrative form are based on the average treatment schedules for health centres given in Table 5.1. Since these schedules distinguish only between adults and children (under 5 years old) this is the only age breakdown required, and the rest of the table provides for these to be recorded separately, with a total column on the extreme right.

Repeat visits for administration of a standard treatment prescribed at an earlier contact (injections, dressings, oral medication) or for follow-up are recorded separately on the last page of the record form. **Contacts for preventive services** such as vaccinations, maternal and child health, family planning and medical examinations without illness **are also recorded separately** under other health service contacts at the end of the record form.

The form is extremely easy to use, for the whole record can be kept on one folded sheet of paper, and no writing is required. When a standard treatment is given (or required) the record keeper simply ticks the first available zero opposite that treatment in the column for adults or children, as appropriate. If the patient has several health problems, for example a worm infestation and malaria, and a standard treatment is required for each one, then each one must be recorded separately.

For health problems/standard drug treatments which occur more frequently two or more rows of zeros may be allowed, as shown in Table 6.4 for malaria and acute diarrhoea. (If all the zeros for a particular problem are crossed out they can be used a second time by crossing diagonally in the opposite direction.) The zeros are grouped in fives so that the numbers can be easily totalled at the end of recording.

Table 6.4
Model record form for the middle level (Health Centre)

Name of Health Centre:
Period: Page:

ICD code		Children under 5	Children five y. and older, adults	Total
	I. INFECTIOUS AND PARASITIC DISEASES			
	Bacterial infections and zoonoses			
001	Cholera	00000 00000 00000	00000 00000 00000 00000 00000 00000	
002.0	Typhoid	00000 00000 00000	00000 00000 00000 00000 00000 00000	
004	Bacillary dysentery	00000 00000 00000	00000 00000 00000 00000 00000 00000	
009.2	Acute diarrhoea mild (severity 1)	00000 00000 00000	00000 00000 00000 00000 00000 00000	
	severe (severity 2)	00000 00000 00000	00000 00000 00000 00000 00000 00000	
		00000 00000 00000	00000 00000 00000 00000 00000 00000	
011	Pulmonary tuberculosis	00000 00000 00000	00000 00000 00000 00000 00000 00000	
030	Leprosy	00000 00000 00000	00000 00000 00000 00000 00000 00000	
	Other bacterial infections and zoonoses	00000 00000 00000	00000 00000 00000 00000 00000 00000	
	Viral and chlamydial infections			
052	Chickenpox	00000 00000 00000	00000 00000 00000 00000 00000 00000	
055	Measles: mild (severity 1)	00000 00000 00000	00000 00000 00000 00000 00000 00000	
	severe (severity 2)	00000 00000 00000	00000 00000 00000 00000 00000 00000	
076	Trachoma	00000 00000 00000	00000 00000 00000 00000 00000 00000	
	Other viral and chlamydial infections	00000 00000 00000	00000 00000 00000 00000 00000 00000	
084	**Malaria:** mild	00000 00000 00000	00000 00000 00000 00000 00000 00000	
		00000 00000 00000	00000 00000 00000 00000 00000 00000	
	severe	00000 00000 00000	00000 00000 00000 00000 00000 00000	
	Venereal diseases			
090-7	Syphilis	00000 00000 00000	00000 00000 00000 00000 00000 00000	
098.0	Gonorrhoea: non-resistant	00000 00000 00000	00000 00000 00000 00000 00000 00000	
	restant	00000 00000 00000	00000 00000 00000 00000 00000 00000	
098.4	Ophthalmia neonatorum	00000 00000 00000		
	Other venereal diseases	00000 00000 00000	00000 00000 00000 00000 00000 00000	
	Fungal infections			
110	Fungal skin infections	00000 00000 00000	00000 00000 00000 00000 00000 00000	
112.1	Candidiasis, vaginal	00000 00000 00000	00000 00000 00000 00000 00000 00000	
	Other fungal infections	00000 00000 00000	00000 00000 00000 00000 00000 00000	
	Helminthic infections			
120.0	Schistosomiasis haematobia	00000 00000 00000	00000 00000 00000 00000 00000 00000	
120.1	Schistosomiasis mansoni	00000 00000 00000	00000 00000 00000 00000 00000 00000	
120.2	Schistosomiasis japonica	00000 00000 00000	00000 00000 00000 00000 00000 00000	
123.3	Taeniasis (tapeworm)	00000 00000 00000	00000 00000 00000 00000 00000 00000	
125.3	Onchocerciasis mild (severity 1)	00000 00000 00000	00000 00000 00000 00000 00000 00000	
	severe (severity 2)	00000 00000 00000	00000 00000 00000 00000 00000 00000	
125	Other filaria	00000 00000 00000	00000 00000 00000 00000 00000 00000	
126	Ancylostomiasis (hookworm)	00000 00000 00000	00000 00000 00000 00000 00000 00000	
127.0	Ascariasis (roundworm)	00000 00000 00000	00000 00000 00000 00000 00000 00000	
	Other helminthic infections	00000 00000 00000	00000 00000 00000 00000 00000 00000	
	Other parasitic infections			
131.0	Trichomoniasis, vaginal	00000 00000 00000	00000 00000 00000 00000 00000 00000	
132	Pediculosis (lice)	00000 00000 00000	00000 00000 00000 00000 00000 00000	
133.0	Scabies	00000 00000 00000	00000 00000 00000 00000 00000 00000	
	Other parasitic infections	00000 00000 00000	00000 00000 00000 00000 00000 00000	

continued

Table 6.4 (continued)

ICD code		Children under 5			Children five y. and older, adults						Total
	III. ENDOCRINE, NUTRITIONAL AND METABOLIC DISORDERS										
250	Diabetes mellitus:	00000	00000	00000	00000	00000	00000	00000	00000	00000	
	non insulin dependent	00000	00000	00000	00000	00000	00000	00000	00000	00000	
	Insulin dependent	00000	00000	00000	00000	00000	00000	00000	00000	00000	
260-3	Malnutrition	00000	00000	00000	00000	00000	00000	00000	00000	00000	
264	Vitamin A deficiency, xerophthalmia	00000	00000	00000	00000	00000	00000	00000	00000	00000	
265-9	Other vitamin deficiency	00000	00000	00000	00000	00000	00000	00000	00000	00000	
	Other endocr. nutr. and metab. disorders	00000	00000	00000	00000	00000	00000	00000	00000	00000	
	IV. DISEASES OF BLOOD AND BLOODFORMING ORGANS										
280	Iron deficiency anaemia	00000	00000	00000	00000	00000	00000	00000	00000	00000	
282.5	Sickle cell disease	00000	00000	00000	00000	00000	00000	00000	00000	00000	
	Other diseases of blood and blf.organs	00000	00000	00000	00000	00000	00000	00000	00000	00000	
	V. MENTAL DISORDERS										
290-9	Psychosis	00000	00000	00000	00000	00000	00000	00000	00000	00000	
300.0	Anxiety neurosis	00000	00000	00000	00000	00000	00000	00000	00000	00000	
300.4	Depressive neurosis	00000	00000	00000	00000	00000	00000	00000	00000	00000	
	Other mental disorders	00000	00000	00000	00000	00000	00000	00000	00000	00000	
	VI. DISEASES OF THE NERVOUS SYSTEM AND SENSE ORGANS										
345.0	Petit-mal epilepsy	00000	00000	00000	00000	00000	00000	00000	00000	00000	
345.1	Grand-mal epilepsy	00000	00000	00000	00000	00000	00000	00000	00000	00000	
345.3	Status epilepticus	00000	00000	00000	00000	00000	00000	00000	00000	00000	
372.0	Conjunctivitis	00000	00000	00000	00000	00000	00000	00000	00000	00000	
380.1	Otitis externa	00000	00000	00000	00000	00000	00000	00000	00000	00000	
381-2	Otitis media: mild (severity 1)	00000	00000	00000	00000	00000	00000	00000	00000	00000	
	severe (severity 2)	00000	00000	00000	00000	00000	00000	00000	00000	00000	
	Other diseases of NS and sense organs	00000	00000	00000	00000	00000	00000	00000	00000	00000	
	VII. DISEASES OF THE CIRCULATORY SYSTEM										
390-8	Rheumatic heart disease	00000	00000	00000	00000	00000	00000	00000	00000	00000	
401-5	Hypertension	00000	00000	00000	00000	00000	00000	00000	00000	00000	
410-4	Ischaemic heart disease	00000	00000	00000	00000	00000	00000	00000	00000	00000	
455	Haemorrhoids	00000	00000	00000	00000	00000	00000	00000	00000	00000	
459.0	Shock	00000	00000	00000	00000	00000	00000	00000	00000	00000	
	Other diseases of circulatory system	00000	00000	00000	00000	00000	00000	00000	00000	00000	
	VIII DISEASES OF THE RESPIRATORY SYSTEM										
460	Common cold, catarrh, sore throat	00000	00000	00000	00000	00000	00000	00000	00000	00000	
		00000	00000	00000	00000	00000	00000	00000	00000	00000	
463	Tonsillitis (bacterial)	00000	00000	00000	00000	00000	00000	00000	00000	00000	
465	Acute bronchitis	00000	00000	00000	00000	00000	00000	00000	00000	00000	
		00000	00000	00000	00000	00000	00000	00000	00000	00000	
480-6	Pneumonia: mild (severity 1)	00000	00000	00000	00000	00000	00000	00000	00000	00000	
	severe (severity 2)	00000	00000	00000	00000	00000	00000	00000	00000	00000	
491	Chronic bronchitis, emphysema	00000	00000	00000	00000	00000	00000	00000	00000	00000	
493	Asthma: mild (severity 1)	00000	00000	00000	00000	00000	00000	00000	00000	00000	
	acute attack (severity 2)	00000	00000	00000	00000	00000	00000	00000	00000	00000	
	Other diseases of the respiratory system	00000	00000	00000	00000	00000	00000	00000	00000	00000	

continued

Table 6.4 (continued)

ICD code		Children under 5			Children five y. and older, adults						Total
	IX. DISEASES OF THE DIGESTIVE SYSTEM										
521.0	Caries, toothache	00000	00000	00000	00000	00000	00000	00000	00000	00000	
522.5	Dental abscess	00000	00000	00000	00000	00000	00000	00000	00000	00000	
528	Mouth sores	00000	00000	00000	00000	00000	00000	00000	00000	00000	
535-6	Gastritis, heartburn, indigestion	00000	00000	00000	00000	00000	00000	00000	00000	00000	
564	Constipation	00000	00000	00000	00000	00000	00000	00000	00000	00000	
	Other diseases of the digestive system	00000	00000	00000	00000	00000	00000	00000	00000	00000	
	X. DISEASES OF THE GENITO URINARY SYSTEM										
595	Cystitis: severity 1	00000	00000	00000	00000	00000	00000	00000	00000	00000	
	severity 2	00000	00000	00000	00000	00000	00000	00000	00000	00000	
614	Pelvic inflammatory disease	00000	00000	00000	00000	00000	00000	00000	00000	00000	
	Other diseases of gen.-urinary system	00000	00000	00000	00000	00000	00000	00000	00000	00000	
	XI. COMPLICATIONS OF PREGNANCY, CHILDBIRTH AND PUERPERIUM										
634-8	Abortion				00000	00000	00000	00000	00000	00000	
650	Normal delivery				00000	00000	00000	00000	00000	00000	
660-5	Abnormal delivery				00000	00000	00000	00000	00000	00000	
666	Postpartum haemorrhage				00000	00000	00000	00000	00000	00000	
670	Major puerperal infection				00000	00000	00000	00000	00000	00000	
675	Mastitis, breast abscess				00000	00000	00000	00000	00000	00000	
	Other complications				00000	00000	00000	00000	00000	00000	
	XII. DISEASES OF THE SKIN AND SUBCUTANEOUS TISSUE										
680-2	Boil, abscess	00000	00000	00000	00000	00000	00000	00000	00000	00000	
684	Bacterial skin infection	00000	00000	00000	00000	00000	00000	00000	00000	00000	
691.8	Eczema	00000	00000	00000	00000	00000	00000	00000	00000	00000	
692	Skin allergy	00000	00000	00000	00000	00000	00000	00000	00000	00000	
698	Itching	00000	00000	00000	00000	00000	00000	00000	00000	00000	
707.9	Chronic ulcer, tropical ulcer	00000	00000	00000	00000	00000	00000	00000	00000	00000	
	Other diseases of the skin	00000	00000	00000	00000	00000	00000	00000	00000	00000	
	XIII. DISEASES OF THE MUSCULOSKELETAL SYSTEM AND CONNECTIVE TISSSUE										
714-6	Arthritis and arthrosis	00000	00000	00000	00000	00000	00000	00000	00000	00000	
724	Backpain, lumbago	00000	00000	00000	00000	00000	00000	00000	00000	00000	
728.0	Pyomyositis	00000	00000	00000	00000	00000	00000	00000	00000	00000	
	Other diseases of the MS system	00000	00000	00000	00000	00000	00000	00000	00000	00000	
	XVI. SYMPTOMS, SIGNS AND ILL-DEFINED CONDITIONS										
780.3	Convulsions, febrile	00000	00000	00000	00000	00000	00000	00000	00000	00000	
780.5	Insomnia	00000	00000	00000	00000	00000	00000	00000	00000	00000	
780.6	Fever NEC	00000	00000	00000	00000	00000	00000	00000	00000	00000	
		00000	00000	00000	00000	00000	00000	00000	00000	00000	
780.7	Malaise, fatigue NEC	00000	00000	00000	00000	00000	00000	00000	00000	00000	
		00000	00000	00000	00000	00000	00000	00000	00000	00000	
784	Headache NEC	00000	00000	00000	00000	00000	00000	00000	00000	00000	
		00000	00000	00000	00000	00000	00000	00000	00000	00000	
786.2	Cough NEC	00000	00000	00000	00000	00000	00000	00000	00000	00000	
		00000	00000	00000	00000	00000	00000	00000	00000	00000	
787	Vomiting	00000	00000	00000	00000	00000	00000	00000	00000	00000	
788.0	Renal colic	00000	00000	00000	00000	00000	00000	00000	00000	00000	
789.0	Abdominal pain NEC	00000	00000	00000	00000	00000	00000	00000	00000	00000	

continued

Table 6.4 (continued)

ICD code		Children under 5	Children five y. and older, adults	Total
	XVII. INJURY AND POISONING			
800-29	Fractures	00000 00000 00000	00000 00000 00000 00000 00000 00000	
830-9	Dislocations	00000 00000 00000	00000 00000 00000 00000 00000 00000	
840-8	Sprains and strains	00000 00000 00000	00000 00000 00000 00000 00000 00000	
850-4	Intracranial injury, concussion	00000 00000 00000	00000 00000 00000 00000 00000 00000	
870-9	Open wound, laceration, major cut	00000 00000 00000	00000 00000 00000 00000 00000 00000	
879.9	Complicated wound, animal or human bite	00000 00000 00000	00000 00000 00000 00000 00000 00000	
910-19	Superficial injury, bruise, minor cut	00000 00000 00000	00000 00000 00000 00000 00000 00000	
		00000 00000 00000	00000 00000 00000 00000 00000 00000	
930	Foreign body in eye	00000 00000 00000	00000 00000 00000 00000 00000 00000	
940-9	Burns	00000 00000 00000	00000 00000 00000 00000 00000 00000	
960-79	Poisoning	00000 00000 00000	00000 00000 00000 00000 00000 00000	
989.5	Snake bite, other stings and bites	00000 00000 00000	00000 00000 00000 00000 00000 00000	
995.0	Anaphylactic shock	00000 00000 00000	00000 00000 00000 00000 00000 00000	
	Other injury or poisoning	00000 00000 00000	00000 00000 00000 00000 00000 00000	
	Total	Children under 5	Children five y. and older, adults	
				Total
	REPEAT VISITS FOR THE SAME HEALTH PROBLEM			------
	Injections	00000 00000 00000	00000 00000 00000 00000 00000 00000	
		00000 00000 00000	00000 00000 00000 00000 00000 00000	
	Dressings	00000 00000 00000	00000 00000 00000 00000 00000 00000	
		00000 00000 00000	00000 00000 00000 00000 00000 00000	
	Oral medication	00000 00000 00000	00000 00000 00000 00000 00000 00000	
		00000 00000 00000	00000 00000 00000 00000 00000 00000	
	Follow-up visit	00000 00000 00000	00000 00000 00000 00000 00000 00000	
		00000 00000 00000	00000 00000 00000 00000 00000 00000	
	OTHER HEALTH SERVICE CONTACTS			
V03-07	Vaccinations	00000 00000 00000 00000	00000 00000 00000 00000 00000 00000	
		00000 00000 00000 00000	00000 00000 00000 00000 00000 00000	
		00000 00000 00000 00000	00000 00000 00000 00000 00000 00000	
V20	Under-five preventive care	00000 00000 00000 00000	00000 00000 00000 00000 00000 00000	
		00000 00000 00000 00000	00000 00000 00000 00000 00000 00000	
		00000 00000 00000 00000	00000 00000 00000 00000 00000 00000	
V22-3	Antenatal care	00000 00000 00000 00000	00000 00000 00000 00000 00000 00000	
		00000 00000 00000 00000	00000 00000 00000 00000 00000 00000	
V25	Family planning, contraception	00000 00000 00000 00000	00000 00000 00000 00000 00000 00000	
		00000 00000 00000 00000	00000 00000 00000 00000 00000 00000	
V70	Medical examination, no disease	00000 00000 00000 00000	00000 00000 00000 00000 00000 00000	
		00000 00000 00000 00000	00000 00000 00000 00000 00000 00000	

EXAMPLE:

Table 6.5 shows a shorter record form for the village health worker level of care (based on the health problems decided to be treatable at this level in Table 4.2) completed with illustrative data.

A look at a few lines of the record form will show how it is used. In the sample period one standard treatment for iron deficiency anaemia was required for a child, and the record keeper has ticked the first zero opposite this health problem in the column for children. There were also 2 treatment episodes for adults and the first two zeros in the column for adults have been ticked.

For some health problems there were still more treatment episodes to record after all the zeros had been ticked. For example, there were 91 treatment episodes for malaria in adults. The record keeper ticked a zero each until all 60 zeros were ticked. He then returned to the first zero and started again, this time crossing them out in the opposite direction. A tick therefore shows one treatment episode or one contact, and a cross means two contacts.

Repeat visits for the administration of treatments prescribed at earlier visits and for follow-up are recorded in the second part of the form. In Table 6.5 we see, for example, that 7 children and 17 adults returned for injections, and 11 children and 25 adults returned for dressings.

Contacts for preventive services, without treatment are similarly recorded in the third part of the record form.

At the end of the sample period, the number of contacts in each category is added up and recorded in the total columns. In this case we see there 495 treatment episodes in all (150 for children and 345 for adults) plus 88 repeat visits making 583 curative contacts. There were also 296 preventive contacts, bringing the total number of contacts to 879.

Once the results are available from all the facilities in the sample they must of course be consolidated, as already described in Table 6.3 and scaled up using the appropriate multiplying factor. Table 6.6 shows some imaginary results. Both absolute figures (Columns 3, 4 and 5) and rates per 1,000 treatment episodes (Columns 6, 7 and 8) are shown. The rates allow comparisons to be made with other data. These will be used in the examples and exercises in Module 7.

Table 6.5
Model recording form for the community health worker

Name....... ....   Location.............. ....

ICD Code	Health problem	Children under 5	Total	Children five and over, & adults	Total	TOTAL ALL
009.2	Acute diarrhoea		30		32	62
084	Malaria (severity 1)		23		91	114
127.0	Ascariasis (roundworm)		30		76	106
132	Pediculosis (lice)		5		10	15
133.0	Scabies		2		5	7
280	Iron deficiency anaemia		1		2	3
372.0	Conjunctivitis		9		7	16
460	Common cold		10		12	22
521.0	Caries, toothache		6		17	23
535-6	Gastritis, heartburn, indigestion	00000 00000 00000			11	11
564.0	Constipation		4		8	12
595	Cystitis	00000 00000 00000			6	6
680-2	Boil, abscess		1		2	3
684	Impetigo, bacterial skin infection		1		2	3
714-6	Chronic arthritis and arthrosis	00000 00000 00000			4	4
724	Back-pain, lumbago	00000 00000 00000			2	2
780.6	Fever NEC		9		6	15
780.7	Malaise, fatigue NEC		3		5	8
784	Headache NEC		1		11	12
786.2	Cough NEC		9		13	22
789.0	Abdominal pain NEC		2		5	7
840-8	Sprains and strains		1		3	4
910-19	Superficial injury, bruise, cut		1		11	12
940-9	Burns		2		4	6
		SUB TOTAL:	150	SUB TOTAL:	345	495
REPEAT VISITS FOR SAME HEALTH PROBLEM						
	Injections		7		17	24
	Dressings		11		25	36
	Oral medication		5		11	16
	Follow-up visit		4		8	12
		SUB TOTAL:	27	SUB TOTAL:	61	88
OTHER HEALTH SERVICE CONTACTS						
V03-07	Vaccinations		60		17	77
V20	Under-five preventive care		58			58
V22-3	Antenatal care				70	70
V25	Family planning, contraception				86	86
V70	Medical examination, no disease	00000 00000 00000			5	5
		SUB TOTAL :	118	SUB TOTAL:	178	296
		GRAND TOTAL:	295	GRAND TOTAL:	584	879

Table 6.6
Total treatment episodes and other contacts by community health workers

ICD Code	Health problem	Children	Adults	TOTAL	Children 0/00	Adults 0/00	TOTAL 0/00
009.2	Acute diarrhoea:						
	Severity 1	18000	25200	43200	51.37	38.49	42.98
	Severity 2	14400	10800	25200	41.10	16.50	25.07
084	Malaria (severity 1)	27600	65520	93120	78.77	100.07	92.65
127.0	Ascariasis (roundworm)	36000	91200	127200	102.74	139.30	126.55
132	Pediculosis (lice)	6000	12000	18000	17.12	18.33	17.91
133.0	Scabies	2400	6000	8400	6.85	9.16	8.36
280	Iron deficiency anaemia	1200	2400	3600	3.42	3.67	3.58
372.0	Conjunctivitis	10800	8400	19200	30.82	12.83	19.10
460	Common cold	12000	14400	26400	34.25	21.99	26.27
521.0	Caries, toothache	7200	20400	27600	20.55	31.16	27.46
535-6	Gastritis, heartburn, indigestion	0	13200	13200	0.00	20.16	13.13
564.0	Constipation	4800	9600	14400	13.70	14.66	14.33
595	Cystitis:						
	Severity 1	0	4800	4800	0.00	7.33	4.78
	Severity 2	0	2400	2400	0.00	3.67	2.39
680-2	Boil, abscess	1200	2400	3600	3.42	3.67	3.58
684	Impetigo, bacterial skin infection	1200	2400	3600	3.42	3.67	3.58
714-6	Chronic arthritis and arthrosis	0	4800	4800	0.00	7.33	4.78
724	Back-pain, lumbago	0	2400	2400	0.00	3.67	2.39
780.6	Fever NEC	10800	7200	18000	30.82	11.00	17.91
780.7	Malaise, fatigue NEC	3600	6000	9600	10.27	9.16	9.55
784.0	Headache NEC	1200	13200	14400	3.42	20.16	14.33
786.2	Cough NEC	10800	15600	26400	30.82	23.83	26.27
789.0	Abdominal pain NEC	2400	6000	8400	6.85	9.16	8.36
840-8	Sprains and strains	1200	3600	4800	3.42	5.50	4.78
910-19	Superficial injury, bruise, cut	1200	13200	14400	3.42	20.16	14.33
940-9	Burns	2400	4800	7200	6.85	7.33	7.16
	TOTAL TREATMENT EPISODES	176400	367920	544320	503.42	561.95	541.55
REPEAT VISIT FOR SAME HEALTH PROBLEM							
	Injections	8400	20400	28800	23.97	31.16	28.65
	Dressings	13200	30000	43200	37.67	45.82	42.98
	Oral medication	6000	13200	19200	17.12	20.16	19.10
	Follow-up visit	4800	9600	14400	13.70	14.66	14.33
	TOTAL REPEAT VISITS	32400	73200	105600	92.47	111.80	105.06
OTHER HEALTH SERVICE CONTACTS							
V03-06	Vaccinations	72000	20400	92400	205.48	31.16	91.93
V20	Under-five preventive care	69600	0	69600	198.63	0.00	69.25
V22-3	Antenatal care	0	84000	84000	0.00	128.30	83.57
V25	Family planning, contraception	0	103200	103200	0.00	157.62	102.67
V70	Medical examination, no disease	0	6000	6000	0.00	9.16	5.97
	TOTAL PREVENTIVE CONTACTS	141600	213600	355200	404.11	326.25	353.39
	GRAND TOTAL	350400	654720	1005120	1000.00	1000.00	1000.00

MODULE 7:

THE PATIENT MORBIDITY/STANDARD TREATMENT METHOD: CALCULATION PROCEDURES

1. INTRODUCTION

So far we have covered tasks 1-11 of the 18 tasks involved in quantifying drug requirements (as summarized in Table 3.1). This module will explain and illustrate tasks 12-15 of the calculation procedures:

Task 12: Calculate the **quantities required** of each drug.

Task 13: Estimate the **cost** of the quantities required.

Task 14: **Reconcile** the quantities to budget, if the budget is inadequate and cannot be increased.

Task 15: Calculate the **average quantity of each drug** required per 1000 **treatment episodes** or per 1000 patient contacts.

2. TASK 12: CALCULATING QUANTITIES REQUIRED OF EACH DRUG

This task involves four steps:

STEP 1: Calculating the total quantity required of each drug for each health problem. To do this, multiply the number of treatment episodes during the year by the quantity of each drug required in that standard treatment.

STEP 2: Reorganize the quantities from step 1 above by drug to obtain the total quantity required of each drug. Where a drug is indicated for more than one standard treatment, add the quantities required for each one, to obtain the total.

STEP 3: Increase the quantities estimated in step two to allow for wastage and losses (damage, date expiry, loss, pilferage and theft).

STEP 4: Convert the quantities from step 3 into the required number of order packs.

STEP 1: Calculate the quantity of each drug required for each health problem.

EXAMPLE:

Suppose we wish to calculate the drug quantities required for village health workers, based on the average standard treatments specified in Table 5.1, and the number of treatment episodes in Table 6.6. The calculation sheet is shown in Table 7.1.

The first health problem (from Table 6.1) is acute diarrhoea (ICD 009.2). Six different standard treatments have been specified for this health problem (Table 5.1) but only severity 1 and severity 2 are to be treated by the village health worker. For severity 1 in children the average treatment is one packet of oral rehydration salts (ORS) to make one litre of fluid. The total number of treatment episodes among children requiring this treatment is 18,000 (from Table 6.6). So 18,000 packets of ORS are needed for these treatment episodes. For severity 2 acute diarrhoea in adults the average standard treatment is 6 packets of ORS and there are 10,800 treatment episodes. So the total quantity required for these treatments is 64,800 packets. The quantities for the other treatments are calculated in the same way.

EXERCISE 7A

1. Table 7.1 shows the number of treatment episodes and the average quantity of each drug required for the standard treatments of the first ten health problems from Table 6.6. The drug quantities required for each standard treatment have been calculated.
   (a) Check that the average drug quantities per standard treatment, given in column 4 are correct (from the treatment schedules in Table 5.1).
   (b) Check that the number of treatment episodes in column 5 are correct (from Table 6.6).
2. In column 2 of Table 7.1 the remaining health problems (from Table 6.6) are listed.
   (a) In column 3, note the drug(s) specified in the standard treatment for each health problem, and in column 4 note the quantity of each drug per standard treatment (from Table 5.1).
   (b) In column 5, note the number of treatment episodes of each standard treatment (from Table 6.6).
3. For each standard treatment multiply the number in column 4 by the corresponding number in column 5 to obtain the total quantity of each drug for each standard treatment.

Check your answers in Table 7.2.

Table 7.1
Calculation sheet for drug quantities by health problem

Abbreviations: S - Severity. A - Adults. C - Children. NEC - Not Elsewhere Classified

1 ICD Code	2 Health problem	3 Standard treatment Drug generic name, dosage form and strength	4 Quantity per standard treatment	5 Number of treatment episodes	6 TOTAL QUANTITY
009.2	Acute diarrhoea				
	S1: A (no dehydration)	oral rehydration salts pkt(1 litre)	2 pkt	25200	50400
	S1: C (no dehydration)	oral rehydration salts pkt(1 litre)	1 pkt	18000	18000
	S2: A (some dehydration)	oral rehydration salts pkt(1 litre)	6 pkt	10800	64800
	S2: C (some dehydration)	oral rehydration salts pkt(1 litre)	2 pkt	14400	28800
084	Malaria (severity 1)				
	S1: A	chloroquine tab 150mg base	10 tab	65520	655200
	S1: C	chloroquine tab 150mg base	2.5 tab	27600	69000
127.0	Ascariasis (roundworm) A+C	mebendazole tab 100 mg	6 tab	127200	763200
132	Pediculosis (lice) A+C	lindane cream 1% 25 g	1 tube	18000	18000
133.0	Scabies A+C	benzylbenzoate lot 25% (g)	60 ml	8400	504000
280	Iron deficiency anaemia				
	A	ferrous sulfate tab 60 mg iron	84 tab	2400	201600
	C	ferrous sulfate tab 60 mg iron	28 tab	1200	33600
372.0	Conjunctivitis A+C	tetracycline eye oint 1% 5g tube	1 tube	19200	19200
460	Common cold				
	A	paracetamol tab 500 mg	8 tab	14400	115200
	C	paracetamol tab 500 mg	4 tab	12000	48000
521.0	Caries, toothache				
	A	acetylsalicylic acid tab 300 mg	16 tab	20400	326400
	C	paracetamol 500 mg	4 tab	7200	28800
535-6	Gastritis, heartburn and indigestion A+(	aluminium hydroxide tab 500 mg	24 tab	13200	316800
564.0	Constipation				
	A				
	C				
595	Cystitis				
	S1: A				
	S2: A				
	S2: C				
680-2	Boil, abscess				
	A				
	C				
684	Impetigo, bacterial skin infection A+C				
714-6	Arthritis & arthrosis				
724	Back-pain, lumbago A				

continued

Table 7.1 (continued)

ICD Code	Health problem	Standard treatment Drug generic name, dosage form and strength	Quantity per standard treatment	Number of treatment episodes	TOTAL QUANTITY
780.6	Fever NEC				
	A				
	C				
780.7	Malaise, fatigue NEC				
784.0	Headache NEC				
	A				
	C				
786.2	Cough NEC				
	A				
	C				
789.0	Abdominal pain NEC				
	A				
	C				
840-8	Sprains and strains				
	A				
	C				
910-19	Superficial injury, bruise, cut A+C				
940-9	Burns				
	A				
	C				
	TOTAL TREATMENT EPISODES				
REPEAT VISITS FOR SAME HEALTH PROBLEM					
	Injections				
	A			20400	
	C			8400	
	Dressings				
	A			30000	
	C			13200	
	Oral medication				
	A			13200	
	C			6000	
	Follow-up visit				
	A			9600	
	C			4800	
	TOTAL REPEAT VISITS			105600	
OTHER HEALTH SERVICE CONTACTS					
V03-06	Vaccinations				
	A			20400	
	C			72000	
V20	Under-five preventive care				
	C			69600	

Table 7.1 (continued)

ICD Code	Health problem	Standard treatment Drug generic name, dosage form and strength	Quantity per standard treatment	Number of treatment episodes	TOTAL QUANTITY
V22-3	Antenatal care				
	A			84000	
V25	Family planning, contraception				
	A			103200	
V70	Medical examination, no illness				
	A			6000	
	C			0	
	TOTAL PREVENTIVE CONTACTS			355200	
	GRAND TOTAL				

Table 7.2
Calculation sheet for drug quantities by health problem (completed)

Abbreviations: S - Severity. A - Adults. C - Children. NEC - Not Elsewhere Classified

1 ICD Code	2 Health problem	3 Standard treatment Drug generic name, dosage form and strength	4 Quantity: per standard treatment	5 Number of treatment episodes	6 TOTAL QUANTITY
009.2	Acute diarrhoea				
	S1: A (no dehydration)	oral rehydration salts pkt(1 litre)	2 pkt	25200	50400
	S1: C (no dehydration)	oral rehydration salts pkt(1 litre)	1 pkt	18000	18000
	S2: A (some dehydration)	oral rehydration salts pkt(1 litre)	6 pkt	10800	64800
	S2: C (some dehydration)	oral rehydration salts pkt(1 litre)	2 pkt	14400	28800
084	Malaria (severity 1)				
	S1: A	chloroquine tab 150mg base	10 tab	65520	655200
	S1: C	chloroquine tab 150mg base	2.5 tab	27600	69000
127.0	Ascariasis (roundworm) A+C	mebendazole tab 100 mg	6 tab	127200	763200
132	Pediculosis (lice) A+C	lindane cream 1% 25 g	1 tub	18000	18000
133.0	Scabies A+C	benzylbenzoate lot 25% (g)	60 ml	8400	504000
280	Iron deficiency anaemia				
	A	ferrous sulfate tab 60 mg iron	84 tab	2400	201600
	C	ferrous sulfate tab 60 mg iron	28 tab	1200	33600
372.0	Conjunctivitis A+C	tetracycline eye oint 1% 5g tube	1 tube	19200	19200
460	Common cold				
	A	paracetamol tab 500 mg	8 tab	14400	115200
	C	paracetamol tab 500 mg	4 tab	12000	48000
521.0	Caries, toothache				
	A	acetylsalicylic acid tab 300 mg	16 tab	20400	326400
	C	paracetamol 500 mg	4 tab	7200	28800
535-6	Gastritis, heartburn and indigestion A+C	aluminium hydroxide tab 500 mg	24 tab	13200	316800
564.0	Constipation				
	A	senna tab 7.5 mg sennosides	2 tab	9600	19200
	C	senna tab 7.5 mg sennosides	0.5 tab	4800	2400
595	Cystitis				
	S1: A	sulfamethoxazole & trimethoprim tab 400 mg & 80 mg	4 tab	4800	19200
		paracetamol tab 500 mg	16 tab	4800	76800
	S2: A	sulfamethoxazole & trimethoprim tab 400 mg & 80 mg	40 tab	2400	96000
	S1: C and S2: C: not applicable	paracetamol tab 500 mg	16 tab	"	38400
	S2: C			0	
680-2	Boil, abscess				
	A	procaine benzylpenicillin 3 MU	0.33 vial	2400	792
		phenoxymethylpenicillin tab 250 mg	40 tab	"	96000
		paracetamol tab 500 mg	8 tab	"	19200
	C	procaine benzylpenicillin 3 MU	0.1 vial	1200	120
		phenoxymethylpenicillin tab 250 mg	10 tab	"	12000
		paracetamol tab 500 mg	2 tab	"	2400
684	Impetigo, bacterial skin infection A+C	neomycin/bacitracin oin (20 g)	1 tube	3600	3600
714-6	Arthritis & arthrosis	acetylsalicylic acid tab 300 mg	40 tab	4800	192000
724	Back-pain, lumbago A	acetylsalicylic acid tab 300 mg	40 tab	2400	96000

continued

Table 7.2 (continued)

ICD Code	Health problem	Standard treatment Drug generic name, dosage form and strength	Quantity: per standard treatment	Number of treatment episodes	TOTAL QUANTITY
780.6	Fever NEC				
	A	paracetamol tab 500 mg	8 tab	7200	57600
	C	paracetamol tab 500 mg	2 tab	10800	21600
780.7	Malaise, fatigue NEC	no drug		9600	0
784.0	Headache NEC				
	A	acetylsalicylic acid tab 300 mg	8 tab	13200	105600
	C	paracetamol tab 500 mg	2 tab	1200	2400
786.2	Cough NEC				
	A	chlorphenamine tab 4 mg	6 tab	15600	93600
	C	chlorphenamine tab 4 mg	3 tab	10800	32400
789.0	Abdominal pain NEC				
	A	acetylsalicylic acid tab 300 mg	8 tab	6000	48000
	C	paracetamol tab 500 mg	2 tab	2400	4800
840-8	Sprains and strains				
	A	acetylsalicylic acid tab 300 mg	8 tab	3600	28800
	C	paracetamol tab 500 mg	2 tab	1200	2400
910-19	Superficial injury, bruise, cut A+C	chlorhexidine sol conc 5 % (ml)	1 ml	14400	14400
940-9	Burns				
	A	chlorhexidine sol conc 5 % (ml)	1 ml	4800	4800
		acetylsalicylic acid tab 300 mg	8 tab	*	38400
	C	chlorhexidine sol conc 5 % (ml)	1 ml	2400	2400
		paracetamol tab 500 mg	2 tab	*	4800
	TOTAL TREATMENT EPISODES			544320	
REPEAT VISITS FOR SAME HEALTH PROBLEM					
	Injections	The drug quantities needed for these repeat visits are included in the quantities per treatment episode calculated in the first section of the table.			
	A			20400	
	C			8400	
	Dressings				
	A			30000	
	C			13200	
	Oral medication				
	A			13200	
	C			6000	
	Follow-up visit				
	A			9600	
	C			4800	
	TOTAL REPEAT VISITS			105600	
OTHER HEALTH SERVICE CONTACTS					
V03-06	Vaccinations	Illustrative calculations have not been done for these contacts.			
	A			20400	
	C			72000	
V20	Under-five preventive care				
	C			69600	

continued

Table 7.2 (continued)

ICD Code	Health problem	Standard treatment Drug generic name, dosage form and strength	Quantity per standard treatment	Number of treatment episodes	TOTAL QUANTITY
V22-3	Antenatal care				
	A			84000	
V25	Family planning, contraception				
	A			103200	
V70	Medical examination, no illness				
	A			6000	
	C			0	
	TOTAL PREVENTIVE CONTACTS			355200	
	GRAND TOTAL			1005120	

STEP 2: Reorganise the quantities from step 1 by drug, to obtain the total quantity required of each drug.

We now have the quantity of each drug required for each health problem. However, since many drugs are used for more than one standard treatment, we need to reorganize the results from Table 7.2 by drug. The calculation sheet for this is shown in Table 7.3.

EXAMPLE:

Taking the drugs in alphabetical order, the first one is acetylsalicylic acid tablets 300 mg. Reading through Table 7.2, this drug is used in seven standard treatments.

521.0	*Caries and toothache (Adults)*
714-6	*Chronic arthritis and arthrosis (Adults)*
724	*Back pain and lumbago (Adults)*
784	*Headache (Adults)*
789	*Abdominal pain (Adults)*
840-8	*Sprains and strains (Adults)*
940-9	*Burns (Adults)*

The code numbers of the health problems (and the severity and age group) are noted in Table 7.3, column 3, and the drug quantities are noted in column 4. As each one is noted, it is ticked off in Table 7.2.

(The code numbers are recorded so that the quantities can still be related to the health problems for which they are required, and to make it easier to check that nothing has been omitted.)

EXERCISE 7B

Columns 3 and 4 of Table 7.3 have been completed for the first eleven drugs in alphabetical order.

1. Read through Table 7.2 for each of these drugs, and check that all the quantities for each one have been noted in Table 7.3.

2. For the remaining drugs on page 2 of Table 7.3 complete columns 3 and 4. Check your answers in Table 7.4.

Table 7.3
Calculation sheet for total quantities of each drug

1 Drug code number	2 Drug generic name, dosage form and strength	3 ICD code of health problem for which indicated & severity & age group	4 Total quantity for all standard treatments (in counting units)	5 Total quantity including allowance for wastage & loss	6 Order pack size = (number of units / pack)	7 Number of packs required (rounded to the nearest whole number)
	acetylsalicylic acid tab 300 mg	521.0 A	326400			
		714-6 A	192000			
		724 A	96000			
		784 A	105600			
		789 A	48000			
		840-8 A	28800			
		940-9 A	38400			
		TOTAL	835200 tab			
	aluminium hydroxide tab 500 mg	535-6 A+C	316800 tab			
	benzyl benzoate lot 25% (g)	133.0 A+C	504000 ml			
	chlorhexidine sol conc 5% (ml)	910-19 A+C	14400			
		940-9 A	4800			
		940-9 C	2400			
		TOTAL	21600 ml			
	chloroquine tab 150 mg base	084 S1 A	655200			
		084 S1 C	69000			
		TOTAL	724200 tab			
	chlorphenamine tab 4 mg	786.2 A	93600			
		786.2 C	32400			
		TOTAL	126000 tab			
	ferrous sulfate tab 60 mg iron	280 A	201600			
		280 C	33600			
		TOTAL	235200 tab			
	lindane cream 1% 25 g	132 A+C	18000			
	mebendazole tab 100 mg	127.0 A+C	763200 tab			
	neomycin/bacitracin oin(tube 20 g)	684 A+C	3600 tube			
	oral rehydration salts pkt(1 litre)	009.2 S1: A	50400			
		009.2 S1: C	18000			
		009.2 S2: A	64800			
		009.2 S2: C	28800			
		TOTAL	162000 PKT			

continued

Table 7.3 (continued)

Drug code number	Drug generic name, dosage form and strength	ICD code of health problem for which indicated & severity & age group	Total quantity for all standard treatments (in counting units)	Total quantity including allowance for wastage & loss	Order pack size = (number of units / pack)	Number of packs required (rounded to the nearest whole number)
	paracetamol tab 500 mg					
		TOTAL	tab			
	phenoxymethylpenicillin tab 250 mg					
		TOTAL	tab			
	procaine benzylpenicillin inj 3 MU					
		TOTAL	vial			
	senna tab 7.5 mg sennosides					
		TOTAL	tab			
	sulfamethoxazole & trimethoprim tab 400 mg & 80 mg					
		TOTAL	tab			
	tetracycline eye oint 1% 5 g tube		tube			
	TOTAL COST					

Table 7.4
Calculation sheet for total quantities of each drug (completed)

1 Drug code number	2 Drug generic name, dosage form and strength	3 ICD code of health problem for which indicated & severity & age group	4 Total quantity for all standard treatments (in counting units)	5 Total quantity including allowance for wastage & loss	6 Order pack size = (number of units / pack)	7 Number of packs required (rounded to the nearest whole number)
	acetylsalicylic acid tab 300 mg	521.0 A	326400			
		714-6 A	192000			
		724 A	96000			
		784 A	105600			
		789 A	48000			
		840-8 A	28800			
		940-9 A	38400			
		TOTAL	835200 tab	876960		
	aluminium hydroxide tab 500 mg	535-6 A+C	316800 tab	332640		
	benzyl benzoate lot 25% (g)	133.0 A+C	504000 ml	529200		
	chlorhexidine sol conc 5% (ml)	910-19 A+C	14400			
		940-9 A	4800			
		940-9 C	2400			
		TOTAL	21600 ml	22680		
	chloroquine tab 150 mg base	084 S1 A	655200			
		084 S1 C	69000			
		TOTAL	724200 tab	760410		
	chlorphenamine tab 4 mg	786.2 A	93600			
		786.2 C	32400			
		TOTAL	126000 tab	132300		
	ferrous sulfate tab 60 mg iron	280 A	201600			
		280 C	33600			
		TOTAL	235200 tab	246960		
	lindane cream 1% 25 g	132 A+C	18000	18900		
	mebendazole tab 100 mg	127.0 A+C	763200 tab	801360		
	neomycin/bacitracin oin(tube 20 g)	684 A+C	3600 tube	3780		
	oral rehydration salts pkt(1 litre)	009.2 S1: A	50400			
		009.2 S1: C	18000			
		009.2 S2: A	64800			
		009.2 S2: C	28800			
		TOTAL	162000 PKT	170100		

continued

Table 7.4 (continued)

Drug code number	Drug generic name, dosage form and strength	ICD code of health problem for which indicated & severity & age group	Total quantity for all standard treatments (in counting units)	Total quantity including allowance for wastage & loss	Order pack size = (number of units / pack)	Number of packs required (rounded to the nearest whole number)
	paracetamol tab 500 mg	460 A	115200			
		460 C	48000			
		521.0 C	28800			
		595 S1: A	76800			
		595 S2: A	38400			
		680-2 A	19200			
		680-2 C	2400			
		780.6 A	57600			
		780.6 C	21600			
		784-0 C	2400			
		789.0 C	4800			
		840-8 C	2400			
		940-9 C	4800			
		TOTAL	422400 tab	443520		
	phenoxymethylpenicillin tab 250 mg	680-2 C	96000			
		680-2 A	12000			
		TOTAL	108000 tab	113400		
	procaine benzylpenicillin inj 3 MU	680-2 A	792			
		680-2 C	120			
		TOTAL	912 vial	957.6		
	senna tab 7.5 mg sennosides	564.0 A	19200			
		564.0 C	2400			
		TOTAL	21600 tab	22680		
	sulfamethoxazole & trimethoprim tab 400 mg & 80 mg	595 S1: A	19200			
		595 S2: A	96000			
		TOTAL	115200 tab	120960		
	tetracycline eye oint 1% 5 g tube	372.0 A+C	19200 tube	20160		
	TOTAL COST					

STEP 3: Increase the quantities estimated in step 2 to allow for wastage and losses.

The quantities in Table 7.4 are strictly those required to treat the estimated patient morbidity. In practice, there is also a certain amount of wastage through damage, date expiry, and loss through pilferage and theft. This needs to be allowed for.

EXAMPLE:

In Table 7.4 column 5, all the quantities estimated in column 4 have been increased by 5% as an allowance for wastage and loss.

The above example is of course simplified. In practice it is advisable to make separate **adjustments for each dosage form.** For example, liquid forms in large bottles may be subject to more wastage (through breakages) than solid dosage forms.

Specific adjustments may be needed **for particular drugs or groups of drugs** with higher or lower than average wastage and loss. For example, dapsone tablets for leprosy are less likely to be pilfered than antibiotics or antimalarials.

STEP 4: Convert the quantities from step 3 into the required number of order packs.

The quantities we have are still expressed in counting or prescribing units, but drugs are ordered and delivered in packs. We must therefore translate these quantities into numbers of order packs. To do this we need to know pack size, that is the number of counting units per pack. The number of order packs required is given by the formula:

$$\frac{\text{Total quantity required (in counting units)}}{\text{Pack size (in counting units)}} = \text{Number of order packs}$$

EXAMPLE:

In Table 7.4 the quantity of 300 mg acetylsalicylic acid tablets estimated to be required is 876,960 tablets. Referring back to the drug list in Table 4.8 we find that these tablets are supplied in tins of 1,000 tablets. The number of order packs required is therefore 876,960/1,000 = 877 (the number of packs is rounded up to the next whole number).

EXERCISE 7C:

In Table 7.4 insert the order pack size for each drug (from Table 4.8), in column 6. For each drug, divide the total in column 5 by the corresponding pack size in column 6, to find the number of packs. Note the results in column 7. Round up the answer to the next whole number. Check your answers in Table 7.5.

3. TASK 13: ESTIMATING THE COST OF THE DRUG QUANTITIES REQUIRED

We now know the total number of packs required of each drug, and we are ready to calculate the total cost. The formula for calculating the total cost of each drug is:

Number of packs required x Price per pack = Total cost of each drug

The calculation sheet for this is shown in Table 7.6 (which is simply an extension of Table 7.5).

EXAMPLE:

For each drug we first need to know the total price per pack. These prices were given in the drug list in Table 4.8. They have been transferred to column 8 of Table 7.6 for the first eleven drugs. We see that a 1,000 tablet tin of acetylsalicylic acid costs $ 0.94 and that the 877 tins required would cost $ 824.38. Similarly, 333 tins of aluminium hydroxide at $ 1.00 per tin, each containing 1,000 tablets, would cost $ 333, and so on for the remaining drugs.

EXERCISE 7D

1. On the first page of Table 7.6 check (from Table 4.8) that the price per pack in column 8 is correct for the first eleven drugs.

2. On page 2 of Table 7.6, insert the missing prices per pack in column 8 (from Table 4.8) and calculate the total cost of each drug, noting the answers in column 9. Check your answer in Table 7.7.

Table 7.5
Calculation sheet for total quantities of each drug, number of order packs (completed)

1 Drug code number	2 Drug generic name, dosage form and strength	3 ICD code of health problem for which indicated & severity & age group	4 Total quantity for all standard treatments (in counting units)	5 Total quantity including allowance for wastage & loss	6 Order pack size = (number of units / pack)	7 Number of packs required (rounded to the nearest whole number)
	acetylsalicylic acid tab 300 mg	521.0 A	326400			
		714-6 A	192000			
		724 A	96000			
		784.0 A	105600			
		789 A	48000			
		840-8 A	28800			
		940-9 A	38400			
		TOTAL	835200 tab	876960	1000	877
	aluminium hydroxide tab 500 mg:	535-6 A+C	316800 tab	332640	1000	333
	benzyl benzoate lot 25% (g)	133.0 A+C	504000 ml	529200	1000	529
	chlorhexidine sol conc 5% (ml)	910-19 A+C	14400			
		940-9 A	4800			
		940-9 C	2400			
		TOTAL	21600 ml	22680	100	227
	chloroquine tab 150 mg base	084 S1 A	655200			
		084 S1 C	69000			
		TOTAL	724200 tab	760410	1000	760
	chlorphenamine tab 4 mg	786.2 A	93600			
		786.2 C	32400			
		TOTAL	126000 tab	132300	1000	132
	ferrous sulfate tab 60 mg iron	280 A	201600			
		280 C	33600			
		TOTAL	235200 tab	246960	1000	247
	lindane cream 1% 25 g	132 A+C	18000	18900	100	189
	mebendazole tab 100 mg	127.0 A+C	763200 tab	801360	100	8014
	neomycin/bacitracin oin(tube 20 g)	684 A+C	3600 tube:	3780	1	3780
	oral rehydration salts pkt(1 litre):	009.2 S1: A	50400			
		009.2 S1: C	18000			
		009.2 S2: A	64800			
		009.2 S2: C	28800			
		TOTAL	162000 PKT	170100	1	170100

continued

Table 7.5 (continued)

Drug code number	Drug generic name, dosage form and strength	ICD code of health problem for which indicated & severity & age group	Total quantity for all standard treatments (in counting units)	Total quantity including allowance for wastage & loss	Order pack size = (number of units / pack)	Number of packs required (rounded to the nearest whole number)
	paracetamol tab 500 mg	460 A	115200			
		460 C	48000			
		521.0 C	28800			
		595 S1: A	76800			
		595 S2: A	38400			
		680-2 A	19200			
		680-2 C	2400			
		780.6 A	57600			
		780.6 C	21600			
		784.0 C	2400			
		789.0 C	4800			
		840-8 C	2400			
		940-9 C	4800			
		TOTAL	422400 tab	443520	1000	444
	phenoxymethylpenicillin tab 250 mg	680-2 C	96000			
		680-2 A	12000			
		TOTAL	108000 tab	113400	1000	113
	procaine benzylpenicillin inj 3 MU	680-2 A	792			
		680-2 C	120			
		TOTAL	912 vial	957.6	1	958
	senna tab 7.5 mg sennosides	564.0 A	19200			
		564.0 C	2400			
		TOTAL	21600 tab	22680	100	227
	sulfamethoxazole & trimethoprim tab 400 mg & 80 mg	595 S1:A	19200			
		595 S2:A	96000			
		TOTAL	115200 tab	120960	1000	121
	tetracycline eye oint 1% 5 g tube	372.0 A+C	19200 tube	20160	1	20160
	TOTAL COST					

Table 7.6
Calculation sheet for total quantities of each drug, number of order packs, and cost

1 Drug code number	2 Drug generic name, dosage form and strength	3 ICD code of health problem for which indicated & severity & age group	4 Total quantity for all standard treatments (in counting units)	5 Total quantity including allowance for wastage & loss	6 Order pack size = (number of units /pack)	7 Number of packs required (rounded to the nearest whole number)	8 Price per pack ($)	9 Total cost	10 Percent of total cost
	acetylsalicylic acid tab 300 mg	521.0 A	326400						
		714-6 A	192000						
		724 A	96000						
		784.0 A	105600						
		789 A	48000						
		840-8 A	28800						
		940-9 A	38400						
		TOTAL	835200 tab	876960	1000	877	0.94	824.38	
	aluminium hydroxide tab 500 mg	535-6 A+C	316800 tab	332640	1000	333	1	333	
	benzyl benzoate lot 25% (g)	133.0 A+C	504000 ml	529200	1000	529	1.57	830.53	
	chlorhexidine sol conc 5% (ml)	910-19 A+C	14400						
		940-9 A	4800						
		940-9 C	2400						
		TOTAL	21600 ml	22680	100	227	0.93	211.11	
	chloroquine tab 150 mg base	084 S1 A	655200						
		084 S1 C	69000						
		TOTAL	724200 tab	760410	1000	760	5.95	4522	
	chlorphenamine tab 4 mg	786.2 A	93600						
		786.2 C	32400						
		TOTAL	126000 tab	132300	1000	132	0.88	116.16	
	ferrous sulfate tab 60 mg iron	280 A	201600						
		280 C	33600						
		TOTAL	235200 tab	246960	1000	247	0.82	202.54	
	lindane cream 1% 25 g	132 A+C	18000	18900	100	189	30	5670	
	mebendazole tab 100 mg	127.0 A+C	763200 tab	801360	100	8014	0.61	4888.54	
	neomycin/bacitracin oin(tube 20 g)	684 A+C	3600 tube	3780	1	3780	0.16	604.8	
	oral rehydration salts pkt(1 litre)	009.2 S1: A	50400						
		009.2 S1: C	18000						
		009.2 S2: A	64800						
		009.2 S2: C	28800						
		TOTAL	162000 PKT	170100	1	170100	0.04	6804	

continued

Table 7.6 (continued)

Drug code number	Drug generic name, dosage form and strength	ICD code of health problem for which indicated & severity & age group	Total quantity for all standard treatments (in counting units)	Total quantity including allowance for wastage & loss	Order pack: size = (number of units / pack)	Number of packs required (rounded to the nearest whole number)	Price per pack ($)	Total cost	Percent of total cost
	paracetamol tab 500 mg	460 A	115200						
		460 C	48000						
		521.0 C	28800						
		595 S1: A	76800						
		595 S2: A	38400						
		680-2 A	19200						
		680-2 C	2400						
		780.6 A	57600						
		780.6 C	21600						
		784.0 C	2400						
		789.0 C	4800						
		840-8 C	2400						
		940-9 C	4800						
		TOTAL	422400 tab	443520	1000	444			
	phenoxymethylpenicillin tab 250 mg	680-2 C	96000						
		680-2 A	12000						
		TOTAL	108000 tab	113400	1000	113			
	procaine benzylpenicillin inj 3 MU	680-2 A	792						
		680-2 C	120						
		TOTAL	912 vial:	957.6	1:	958			
	senna tab 7.5 mg sennosides	564.0 A	19200						
		564.0 C	2400						
		TOTAL	21600 tab	22680	100	227			
	sulfamethoxazole & trimethoprim tab 400 mg & 80 mg	595 S1: A	19200						
		595 S2: A	96000						
		TOTAL	115200 tab	120960	1000	121			
	tetracycline eye oint 1% 5 g tube	372.0 A+C	19200 tube	20160	1:	20160			
	TOTAL COST								

Table 7.7
Calculation sheet for total quantities of each drug, number of order packs, and cost (completed)

1 Drug code number	2 Drug generic name, dosage form and strength	3 ICD code of health problem for which indicated & severity & age group	4 Total quantity for all standard treatments (in counting units)	5 Total quantity including allowance for wastage & loss	6 Order: pack size = (number of units / pack)	7 Number of packs required (rounded to the nearest whole number)	8 Price per pack ($)	9 Total cost	10 Percent of total cost
	acetylsalicylic acid tab 300 mg	521.0 A	326400						
		714-6 A	192000						
		724 A	96000						
		784.0 A	105600						
		789 A	48000						
		840-8 A	28800						
		940-9 A	38400						
		TOTAL	835200 tab	876960	1000	877	0.94	824.38	2.63
	aluminium hydroxide tab 500 mg	535-6 A+C:	316800 tab	332640	1000	333	1	333	1.06
	benzyl benzoate lot 25% (g)	133.0 A+C:	504000 ml	529200	1000	529	1.57	830.53	2.65
	chlorhexidine sol conc 5% (ml)	910-19 A+C	14400						
		940-9 A	4800						
		940-9 C	2400						
		TOTAL	21600 ml	22680	100	227	0.93	211.11	0.67
	chloroquine tab 150 mg base	084 S1 A	655200						
		084 S1 C	69000						
		TOTAL	724200 tab	760410	1000	760	5.95	4522	14.45
	chlorphenamine tab 4 mg	786.2 A	93600						
		786.2 C	32400						
		TOTAL	126000 tab	132300	1000	132	0.88	116.16	0.37
	ferrous sulfate tab 60 mg iron	280 A	201600						
		280 C	33600						
		TOTAL	235200 tab	246960	1000	247	0.82	202.54	0.65
	lindane cream 1% 25 g	132 A+C	18000	18900	100	189	30	5670	18.12
	mebendazole tab 100 mg:	127.0 A+C:	763200 tab	801360	100	8014	0.61	4888.54	15.62
	neomycin/bacitracin oin(tube 20 g)	684 A+C	3600 tube	3780	1	3780	0.16	604.8	1.93
	oral rehydration salts pkt(1 litre)	009.2 S1: A	50400						
		009.2 S1: C	18000						
		009.2 S2: A	64800						
		009.2 S2: C	28800						
		TOTAL	162000 PKT	170100	1	170100	0.04	6804	21.75

continued

Table 7.7 continued

Drug code number	Drug generic name, dosage form and strength	ICD code of health problem for which indicated & severity & age group	Total quantity for all standard treatments (in counting units)	Total quantity including allowance for wastage & loss	Order: pack size = (number of units / pack)	Number of packs required (rounded to the nearest whole number)*	Price per pack ($)	Total cost	Percent of total cost
	paracetamol tab 500 mg	460 A	115200						
		460 C	48000						
		521.0 C	28800						
		595 S1: A	76800						
		595 S2: A	38400						
		680-2 A	19200						
		680-2 C	2400						
		780.6 A	57600						
		780.6 C	21600						
		784.0 C	2400						
		789.0 C	4800						
		840-8 C	2400						
		940-9 C	4800						
		TOTAL	422400 tab	443520	1000	444	2.6	1154.4	3.69
	phenoxymethylpenicillin tab 250 mg	680-2 C	96000						
		680-2 A	12000						
		TOTAL	108000 tab	113400	1000	113	7.51	848.63	2.71
	procaine benzylpenicillin inj 3 MU	680-2 A	792						
		680-2 C	120						
		TOTAL	912 vial	957.6	1	958	0.24	229.92	0.73
	senna tab 7.5 mg sennosides	564.0 A	19200						
		564.0 C	2400						
		TOTAL	21600 tab	22680	100	227	2.55	578.85	1.85
	sulfamethoxazole & trimethoprim tab 400 mg & 80 mg	595 S1: A	19200						
		595 S2: A	96000						
		TOTAL	115200 tab	120960	1000	121	17	2057	6.57
	tetracycline eye oint 1% 5 g tube	372.0 A+C	19200 tube	20160	1	20160	0.07	1411.2	4.51
	TOTAL COST							31287.06	100

4. TASK 14: RECONCILING DRUG QUANTITIES TO BUDGET

In ideal circumstances, the budget would be made available to pay for the drugs estimated to be required. In practice, this is generally not the case. Both the budget in national currency, and the foreign exchange allocations, to pay for imports, are likely to be limited. The first step is to make a case for extra budget and to search for extra budgetary funds. If the funds available are still insufficient, then the quantities required must be reviewed and reduced to bring the total order within budget.

A useful tool for doing this is the **VEN system** developed by the State Pharmaceutical Corporation in Sri Lanka. Under such a system all drugs on the essential drug list are classified into one of the following three categories:

V: Vital - drugs which are potentially life saving, which cannot be withdrawn without serious consequences, or which are of major importance in basic health services, especially vaccines and other preventive drugs.

E: Essential - drugs which are effective against less life threatening but nevertheless significant health problems.

N: Non or less essential - drugs for minor or self limiting health problems, or which have a high cost for small extra effectiveness. Table 7.8 shows sample guidelines for determining VEN categories.

Such a classification is not always as easy as it might seem, for drugs for self limiting but frequent problems, such as acetylsalicylic acid or paracetamol for minor pains, are often widely used as placebos, and if not available leave many patients dissatisfied and less likely to return when they have more serious problems.

A second useful tool is an **ABC value analysis.** It is well known from experience, that a relatively small number of drugs generally account for a large proportion of total drug costs. In an ABC analysis, drugs are classified according to their share of total cost:

A: Drugs accounting for a high percentage of cost.

B: Drugs accounting for a medium percentage of cost.

C: Drugs accounting for a low percentage of costs.

These groups help to focus attention on the most important items of cost. The actual cut off points between A, B, and C may be placed wherever they seem most appropriate.

Table 7.8
Sample guidelines for VEN categories

Characteristic of Individual Drugs	Vital (V)	Essential (E)	Non-Essential (N)
Occurrence of Target Condition(s)			
Persons Affected (% of population)	>5%	1-5%	<1%
Persons Diagnosed (cases/100,000 population/year)	200	50-100	50
Persons Treated (frequency target condition seen by health workers)	Moderate to High	Low	Very Low
Severity of Target Condition(s)			
Life Threatening (likely to cause death if untreated)	Possibly	Infrequently	Rarely
Chronic (likely to cause recurrence, relapse, continued disease if untreated)	Possibly	Infrequently	Rarely
Disabling (likely to cause permanent disability if untreated)	Possibly	Infrequently	Rarely
Restricting (likely to cause loss of working and housekeeping time)	Frequently	Occasionally	Infrequently
Therapeutic Effects			
Drug Action	Prevention of Disease, Cure of Disease, Prevention of Complications	Cure of Disease, Prevention or Treatment of Complications	Cure of Self-Limited Disease, Palliative Treatment of Minor Symptoms, Complications
Therapeutic Efficacy	Proven Effective or Probably Effective	Probably Effective	Possibly Effective Unknown, or Proven Ineffective
Cost*			
Average Cost of a Single Course-of-Therapy (acute therapy)	Low	Moderate	High
Average Yearly Cost of Therapy (chronic therapy)	Low	Moderate	High

*Cost considerations may be omitted in assigning VEN categories.
Source: Managing Drug Supply, Boston 1982

EXAMPLE:

The cost of each drug as a percentage of the total is shown in Table 7.9 column 5.

Four drugs each account for over 10% of costs and might be classified as A: oral rehydration salts (21.74%), lindane (18.12%), mebendazole (15.62%) and chloroquine (14.47%). Together they account for 69.48% of costs.

Another two drugs account for 4-10% of cost each: sulfamethoxazole/trimethoprim (6.57%) and tetracycline eye ointment (4.51%). They account for another 11.08% and can be classified as B. The remaining ten drugs account for a total of 19.44% and can be classified C.

The drugs in Table 7.9 have not been classified into VEN categories, but the following example will illustrate the kinds of decisions that might be made in reconciling estimated drug quantities to the available budget.

Table 7.9
Final quantities and cost after reconciliation to budget, and quantities per 1000 treatment episodes

1 Drug generic name, dosage form and strength	2 Number of packs required (rounded to the nearest whole number)	3 Price per pack: ($)	4 Total cost ($)	5 Percent of total cost	6 Final number of packs required adjusted to budget:	7 Pack size (in counting units)	8 TOTAL COST ($)	9 Final quantity (in counting) units)	10 number of counting units per 1000 treatment episodes
acetylsalicylic acid tab 300 mg	877	0.94	824.38	2.63	700	1000	658	700000	1287
aluminium hydroxide tab 500 mg	333	1	333	1.06	84	1000	84	84000	154
benzyl benzoate lot 25% (g)	530	1.57	832.1	2.66	530	1000	832.1	530000	974
chlorhexidine sol conc 5% (ml)	227	0.93	211.11	0.67	227	100	211.11	22700	42
chloroquine tab 150 mg base	761	5.95	4527.95	14.47	761	1000	4527.95	761000	1399
chlorphenamine tab 4 mg	132	0.88	116.16	0.37	132	1000	116.16	132000	243
ferrous sulfate tab 60 mg iron	247	0.82	202.54	0.65	247	100	202.54	24700	45
lindane cream 1%(ml) (tube)	189	30	5670	18.12	100	100	3000	10000	18
mebendazole tab 100 mg	8014	0.61	4888.54	15.62	8014	100	4888.54	801400	1473
neomycin/bacitracin oin(tube 20 g)	3780	0.16	604.8	1.93	3780	1	604.8	3780	7
oral rehydration salts pkt(1 litre)	170100	0.04	6804	21.74	140000	1	5600	140000	257
paracetamol tab 500 mg	444	2.6	1154.4	3.69	350	1000	910	350000	643
phenoxymethylpenicillin tab 250 mg	113	7.51	848.63	2.71	113	1000	848.63	113000	208
procaine benzylpenicillin inj 3 MU	958	0.24	229.92	0.73	958	1	229.92	958	2
senna tab 7.5 mg sennosides	227	2.55	578.85	1.85	114	100	290.7	11400	21
sulfamethoxazole & trimethoprim tab 400 mg & 80 mg	121	17	2057	6.57	121	1000	2057	121000	222
tetracyclin eye oin 1% 5 g tube	20160	0.07	1411.2	4.51	20160	1	1411.2	20160	37
TOTAL COST			31294.58	99.98			26472.65		

Total number of treatment episodes (from Table 6.6) : 544.320

EXAMPLE:

The total cost of the estimated requirements in Table 7.9 is $ 31,294.58. Suppose the available budget were only $ 26,500. We would need to cut the estimated quantities by $ 4,794.58. Looking at the non or less essential items first:

18,900 tubes of lindane cream (for pediculosis-lice) cost $ 5,670.00, or 10.12% of costs. Cutting this to 10,000 tubes reduces the cost to $ 3,000.00,
saving $ 1,417.50

227 packets of senna tablets (for constipation) cost $ 578.85, or only 1.8% of costs, but cutting the order by half to 114 packets is unlikely to involve any major ill-effects, and reduces their cost to $ 290.70,
saving $ 288.15

333 packs of aluminium hydroxide (for indigestion) cost $333, or only 1% of costs, but cutting this symptomatic treatment from a course of 24 tablets to 6 tablets enables the quantity to be reduced to 84 packs at a cost of $ 84.00,
saving $ 249.00

444 tins of paracetamol (for pain in children) cost $ 1,154.40, or 3.7% of costs. Though this drug is not essential, pain in children is often of serious concern to parents, so the quantity is reduced only to 350 tins at a cost of $ 910.00,
saving $ 244.40

877 tins of acetylsalicylic acid tablets (for pain and arthritis in adults) cost $ 824.38, or 2.6% of costs. Cutting this by 20% (as with paracetamol above) makes 700 tins, costing $ 658.00,
saving $ 166.38

Suppose we now turn to the category A drugs which account for high percentages of costs. The largest item is oral rehydration salts (diarrhoea) which accounts for 21.7% of costs. Why is so much ORS required?

Looking back to Table 7.7, we find that the bulk of the 170,100 sachets is used for severity 2 cases. It has been assumed that approximately one third of all diarrhoea cases would be of severity two (5-9% dehydration) and that each of these cases would receive 2 sachets (for a child) and 6 sachets (for an adult). On reflection, the proportion of adults with such dehydration might seem too high for routine circumstances, and the average need of six sachets per adult might be too great. For these reasons the amount of ORS may be reduced by 30,100 (or approximately 18%) reducing the cost from $ 6,804.00 to $ 5,600.00, saving $ 1,204.00

The total savings at this point are $ 4,821.93, and total spending is reduced to $ 26,472.65 which is within the budget of $ 26,500.00.

This example shows that reduction of quantities should start with non- or less essential items. It also shows that a moderate reduction in category A items (percentage-wise) can result in considerable savings in absolute terms. It will be obvious that, if category A items are, in fact, non- or less essential drugs, a reduction in their quantities can be much bigger and can yield considerable savings.

EXERCISE 7E

> Make your own reductions in the drug quantities shown in Table 7.9 to fit a budget of $ 24,000.00, and give your reasons for each reduction.

5. TASK 15: CALCULATING AVERAGE DRUG REQUIREMENTS PER 1,000 TREATMENT EPISODES OR PER 1,000 PATIENT CONTACTS

The purpose of this calculation is to enable drugs to be allocated to individual facilities according to their number of treatment episodes or patient contacts. The formula is:

$$\text{Quantity of each drug per 1,000 treatment episodes} = \frac{\text{Total quantity of each drug}}{\text{total number of treatment episodes of all kinds (in thousands)}}$$

EXAMPLE:

The quantity of each drug per 1,000 treatment episodes is calculated in Table 7.9, column 10.

We know that the drug quantities in column 9 are intended to cover a total of 544,320 treatment episodes (from Table 6.6). Starting with acetylsalicylic acid, the first drug in the list, the total order quantity, 700,000 tablets/544,320 treatment episodes = 1,287 tablets per 1,000 treatment episodes.

For the second drug, aluminium hydroxide, the total order quantity, 84,000 tablets/544,320 treatment episodes = 154 tablets per 1,000 treatment episodes, and so on for each drug.

On the basis of these results a community health worker with a thousand treatment episodes annually would be allocated 1,287 acetylsalicylic acid tablets, 154 aluminium hydroxide tablets, and so on; a CHW with two thousand treatment episodes would receive twice these amounts, and so on proportionately to the number of treatment episodes. In practice, actual deliveries would be made in order packs or, if necessary, fractions of order packs re-packed for distribution.

The same calculation can be done per 1,000 patient contacts if contacts rather than treatment episodes are recorded routinely.

PART III

THE CONSUMPTION METHOD

MODULE 8:

THE ADJUSTED CONSUMPTION METHOD: CALCULATION PROCEDURE

1. INTRODUCTION

The adjusted consumption method estimates drug requirements on the basis of actual drug use per 1,000 patient contacts in a sample of "standard" facilities, where the pattern and level of consumption are considered acceptable. In some cases an adjustment upwards or downwards may be needed for drug quantities where consumption is considered inappropriate.

In other words, the adjusted **consumption** in the "standard" facilities is considered to be a reasonable approximation of the **need** for drugs in other facilities of the same kind. This requires that:

(a) prescribing patterns in the "standard" facilities are considered to be broadly reasonable; and
(b) that the pattern of morbidity treated is representative of the pattern in the rest of the country or region concerned.

When compared with the morbidity method, this method offers less scope for systematic development to improve drug supply and prescribing practice. Its advantages are that it does not require either detailed data on patient morbidity, or standard treatment schedules. However, users of this method should pay particular attention to the fact that any irrational consumption patterns in the "standard" facilities, which are not corrected in the adjustment process, will be included in the drug estimates for all facilities of the type covered by the calculation.

It is important to realize that drug use is not identical to drug need. For example, high consumption of antibiotics because of indiscriminate prescribing, or the use of sophisticated or expensive forms might be interpreted as a need, whereas simpler or cheaper preparations would suffice.

In addition, it must be emphasized that also for the adjusted consumption method to be successful, it is crucial to improve prescribing in order to bring it into line with the drug need estimates. One means to do this is to use standard treatment schedules.

2. METHOD OF CALCULATION

As noted in Table 3.1, steps 1-9 and 13-18 are the same as in the morbidity method. This Module deals with the three tasks 10-12 of the calculation procedure for the consumption method.

Task 10:

Select the "standard" facilities whose consumption is to serve as the norm for the drug quantities to be supplied to all facilities of the same type.

Task 11:

Estimate the number of patient contacts at all facilities of the type for which drug needs are being estimated.

Task 12:

Calculate the average drug use per 1,000 patient contacts and the quantity required of each drug.

3. TASK 10: SELECT THE "STANDARD" FACILITIES WHOSE CONSUMPTION IS TO SERVE AS THE NORM FOR THE DRUG QUANTITIES TO BE SUPPLIED TO ALL FACILITIES OF THE SAME TYPE

This is probably the most crucial decision in the whole procedure. The six criteria listed in Table 8.1 should be applied in selecting the "standard" facilities. Each one is briefly explained below.

Table 8.1
Criteria for selecting "standard" facilities

"Standard" facilities should have:
1. A representative pattern of **morbidity** and patient attendances.
2. Acceptable patterns of rational **prescribing.**
3. Adequate and uninterrupted drug supply.
4. Complete and accurate data on **drug stocks, deliveries and use.**
5. A low level of drug **losses and wastage.**
6. Complete and accurate data on **patient attendances and admissions.**

1. **A representative pattern of morbidity and patient attendances.** The pattern of morbidity in the population served by the "standard" facility and the level of patient attendances should be as representative as possible of the morbidity profile of the region or country for which the estimate is being made. As noted in step one above, if there are significant differences in the morbidity patterns of patients treated by facilities e.g. in urban and rural areas or in different geographical regions of the country, then separate "standard" facilities should be selected to reflect these differences.

2. **Acceptable patterns of rational prescribing.** The prescribing practices in the "standard" facilities should be sufficiently rational to be accepted as an appropriate working norm for all facilities of the type concerned.

   Since this method uses neither detailed patient morbididity data nor standard drug treatment schedules, the assessment of prescribing must largely be based on impressions. However, certain reference points may be used, such as the proportion of injectable drug forms, and the average number of drugs per prescription.

3. **Adequate and uninterrupted drug supply.** The supply of drugs at "standard" facilities should be adequate to meet demand and enable good prescribing practices to be followed. Ideally this means that every drug should be in stock as and when required throughout the period for which consumption is calculated (normally one or two years). In practice, the drug supply may be considered adequate if stock-outs (that is, periods when particular drugs are out of stock) are short, and do not bias patient consultation patterns or prescribing practice. As a working rule the drug supply should be considered inadequate if high priority drugs are out of stock for a total of more than three months during the year.

4. **Complete and accurate data on drug stocks and use.** The "standard" facilities must have complete, accurate and up-to-date data on their drug stocks, deliveries and use. Stock or bin cards are preferable to simple records of drugs used, for information on stocks is essential to check whether there have been stock-outs, how often they occurred, and how long they lasted.

5. **Complete and accurate data on patient attendances.** The "standard" facilities must have complete, accurate and up-to-date data on the total number of patient attendances. For the consumption method, only the total number of out-patient consultations and in-patient admissions is strictly necessary, but it is useful to have more detailed information on the composition of the workload to determine whether the facility concerned has a representative pattern of patient attendances. Examples of useful additional details are: the number of consultations by broad age group, and separate data for preventive consultations (e.g. antenatal controls, vaccinations, family planning visits).

6. **A low level of wastage and losses.** Wastage and losses of drugs through damage, date expiry, and pilferage should be limited, for they are included in the recorded consumption and would distort and exaggerate the estimates if they were too high.

4. TASK 11: ESTIMATE THE NUMBER OF PATIENT CONTACTS AT ALL FACILITIES OF THE TYPE(S) CONCERNED

This task involves two steps:

Step 1: Obtain a list of all the facilities concerned.

Step 2: Assemble from routine statistics the total number of patient contacts at each facility.

If there are out-patient and in-patient contacts, these should be noted, separately. Contacts for preventive care should also be noted separately if possible.

5. TASK 12: CALCULATE THE AVERAGE DRUG USE PER 1,000 PATIENT CONTACTS AND THE QUANTITY REQUIRED OF EACH DRUG

This task involves seven steps:

Step 1: Select the period for which the consumption is to be calculated.

Step 2: Calculate the consumption of each drug.

Step 3: Adjust these quantities for avoidable wastage and losses.

Step 4: Adjust the quantities for stock-outs, if necessary.

Step 5: Calculate the average drug use per 1,000 patient contacts.

Step 6: Consolidate the answers from all the "standard" facilities in the sample.

Step 7: Scale up the answer from the sample to cover all facilities.

STEP 1: Select the period for which consumption is to be calculated.

The simplest and most practical period for which to calculate consumption is one year, so that the morbidity variations of all the seasons are covered. (If data are available, a longer period requires little extra effort and can improve the reliability of the results.) The year or years chosen should be typical in terms of morbidity for the region or country concerned. For example, an epidemic would not only cause high consumption of drugs for the epidemic health problems but also produce an atypical pattern of morbidity per 1,000 patient contacts. If a shorter period than a year is chosen, then be careful to ensure that it is representative of the whole year. For example, it would not be appropriate to take the consumption of three months during the dry season and multiply by four to estimate the full year's consumption.

STEP 2: Calculate the consumption of each drug.

There are two possible methods:

1. Calculation from patient registers - if drug treatments are recorded in patient registers then the quantities dispensed may be added up directly from these registers. This method is reliable only if the records are well kept and complete. It also requires long and time consuming additions where errors may occur.

2. Calculation from stock records in the stores of the health facility, using one of the following methods:

(a) Add up all the quantities issued. This is the simplest method, but it can be tedious if there have been many issues.

(b) Alternatively, use the following formula:

Consumption = Opening Stock + Drugs Received − Closing Stock

Larger facilities will normally record the above data on their own stock or bin cards. For smaller facilities, like village health posts and small health centres, the data will be available in the stock records of the facility supplying the drugs, for example the regional or national pharmaceutical depot. The calculation is demonstrated below using illustrative data for a "standard" hospital.

EXAMPLE:

Suppose the calculation period is one calendar year; deliveries, stocks and issues of drugs are recorded on stock cards; and the first drug on the hospital's essential drug list is lidocaine in 50ml vials, stock number 01200201. The stock card for this drug is shown in Table 8.2. Using method 2(a) we add all the quantities issued during the year shown in the "out" column. The total is 120 vials. This method is quick if there has been a small number of issues, but requires a long addition if there have been many. Alternatively, we may use method 2(b). The stock at 1st January + drugs received during the year - the stock at 31 December = 20 + (60 + 70) - 30 = 120 vials. Method 2 (b) is faster if there is a large number of issues and a small number of drug deliveries. The answer is recorded in the calculation sheet shown in Table 8.6.

(Note: Drug deliveries are from the central medical depot to the main hospital store. Issues are from the main hospital store to the hospital pharmacy. In some hospitals drug deliveries may be made directly to the hospital pharmacy which in turn issues drugs to ward drug cupboards or sub pharmacies.)

Now complete Exercise 8A to check whether you have understood this step in the estimation.

EXERCISE 8A

Calculate the consumption of acetylsalicylic acid tablets for the year using method 2 (a) and 2(b). The stock card is shown in Table 8.2. There are no stock-outs, so no adjustment is needed for this. You may also assume that there was no avoidable wastage or loss, so no adjustment is required for this either.

Check your answer at the foot of page 8.10 and in Table 8.6.

Table 8.2
Illustrative stock cards

DRUG: LIDOCAINE (INJECTABLE) 1% 50ML VIALS

CODE NUMBER: 01200201

DATE 1986		IN	OUT	STOCK
1 Jan	Opening stock			20
5 Jan	From central depot	60		80
18 Jan	To hospital pharmacy		20	60
10 Apr	" "		10	50
6 Jun	" "		10	40
8 Jun	From central depot	70		110
15 Jul	To hospital pharmacy		20	90
20 Aug	" "		20	70
10 Sep	" "		10	60
25 Oct	" "		10	50
10 Nov	" "		10	40
20 Nov	" "		10	30
31 Dec	Closing stock			30

DRUG: ACETYLSALICYLIC ACID TABLETS 300MG

CODE NUMBER: 02100101

DATE 1986		IN	OUT	STOCK
1 Jan	Opening stock			50 000
10 Feb	To hospital pharmacy		20 000	30 000
15 Mar	" "		20 000	10 000
1 Apr	From central depot	80 000		90 000
2 Apr	To hospital pharmacy		10 000	80 000
10 May	" "		20 000	60 000
20 Jun	" "		20 000	40 000
15 Jul	" "		10 000	30 000
1 Aug	From central depot	100 000		130 000
10 Aug	To hospital pharmacy		20 000	110 000
20 Sep	" "		20 000	90 000
10 Oct	From central depot	70 000		160 000
15 Oct	To hospital pharmacy		20 000	140 000
10 Dec	" "		20 000	120 000
31 Dec	Closing stock			120 000

STEP 3: Adjust for avoidable wastage and losses.

A certain percentage of wastage and losses of drugs is unavoidable, but it should not exceed 5-10% in a well run store or pharmacy. In practice, however, some countries are experiencing wastage and losses as high as 30%. The main reasons are: poor stock management (notably excessive order quantities and failing to observe the first in - first out rule leading to wastage through time-expiry); poor storage and careless handling so that drugs are damaged or destroyed; and theft because of poor security. Recorded consumption of drugs should therefore also be adjusted for avoidable wastage and losses using the following formula:

Consumption adjusted for avoidable wastage	=	Recorded consumption	–	Avoidable wastage

EXAMPLE:

Table 8.3 shows the stock-card for injectable procaine benzylpenicillin 3 mega units in 5ml vials. The recorded consumption is 5,800 vials (the total of the out column). Reading down the card we see there have been no stock-outs so no adjustment is needed for this. However, on 14 August we find a total of 800 vials in the "out" column with the explanation "time expired - destroyed". On 1 October we find another entry in the out column for 300 vials "crushed in store". Finally, at the end of the year the closing stock should be 1,000 vials, but the physical inventory shows only 500, so 500 are unaccounted for - and have probably been stolen. It is reasonable to assume that all three items were avoidable. They add up to a total avoidable wastage and loss of 1,600 vials (27.6% of recorded consumption). Adjusted consumption after allowing for avoidable wastage and losses is therefore 5,800-1,600 = 4,200 vials.

The answer is recorded in the calculation sheet shown in Table 8.6.

EXERCISE 8B

Table 8.3 shows the stock-card for sulfadimidine tablets 500mg.

1. What is the recorded consumption for the year?

2. What avoidable wastage and losses have occurred?

3. What is the adjusted consumption after allowing for avoidable wastage and losses?

Check your answer at the foot of page 8.13 and in Table 8.6.

Table 8.3
Illustrative stock cards

DRUG: PROCAINE BENZYLPENICILLIN INJ 3.0 MU

CODE NUMBER: 02100701

DATE 1986		IN	OUT	STOCK
1 Jan	Starting stock			1 800
14 Jan	To hospital pharmacy		600	1 200
5 Feb	From central depot	1 500		2 700
10 Mar	To hospital pharmacy		600	2 100
15 May	" "		600	1 500
10 Jun	From central depot	1 500		3 000
12 Jul	To hospital pharmacy		600	2 400
14 Aug	Time expired/destroyed		800	1 600
10 Sep	To hospital pharmacy		600	1 000
1 Oct	Crushed in store		300	700
18 Nov	To hospital pharmacy		600	100
30 Nov	From central depot	1 500		1 600
15 Dec	To hospital pharmacy		600	1 000
31 Dec	Closing stock			1 000
Unaccounted for			500	
Physically accounted for				500

DRUG: SULFADIMIDINE TABLETS 500 MG

CODE NUMBER: 06320801

DATE 1986		IN	OUT	STOCK
1 Jan	Starting stock			20 000
5 Jan	To hospital pharmacy		8 000	12 000
14 Jan	From central depot	20 000		32 000
15 Mar	To hospital pharmacy		8 000	24 000
12 May	" "		8 000	16 000
10 Jun	Destroyed by damp		7 000	9 000
15 Jun	From central depot	20 000		29 000
8 Jul	To hospital pharmacy		6 000	23 000
14 Sep	" "		5 000	18 000
5 Oct	From central depot	20 000		38 000
20 Nov	Time expired/destroyed		10 000	28 000
22 Nov	To hospital pharmacy		8 000	20 000
28 Dec	" "		7 000	13 000
31 Dec	Closing stock			13 000
Unaccounted for			5 000	
Physically accounted for				8 000

STEP 4: Adjust consumption for stock-outs if necessary.

The consumption method estimates drug requirements on the basis of actual consump tion in "standard" facilities over a given period of time, and relates this consumption t the number of patient consultations and admissions during that period. If a drug ha been out of stock for part of the period, then the consumption recorded applies only t that part of the time when the drug was in stock. For example, if the period for whicl consumption is being calculated is one year, and we find that a given drug was out c stock for three months of that year, then the observed consumption covers only the nin months when the drug was actually available to be prescribed and dispensed to patients.

In practice, relatively short stock-outs of up to one month may be ignored because the are not likely to have a significant effect on estimated drug requirements. For example suppose the estimates are being made from the stock cards of the main store of a hospi tal. When the store issues its last supply of a given drug to the hospital pharmacy th stock cards show a stock-out.

However, in reality, the hospital still has a limited stock of the drug until the last issu is actually used up. The quantities issued and the length of time between issues from th main store give a reasonable idea of how long the drug will still be available in the phar macy after the last issue.

For stock-outs longer than 30 days (1 month) an adjustment should be made. The for mula for making this correction is:

$$\text{Recorded consumption} \times \frac{\text{Period in calculation (in days, weeks or months)}}{\text{Period in stock (in days, weeks or months)}} = \text{Consumption adjusted for stock outs}$$

Answer to exercise 8A: consumption of acetylsalicylic acid tablets:
Method 2(a) total quantity issued = the total in the "out" column = 180,000 tablets.
Method 2(b) opening stock + deliveries - closing stock = 50,000 + (80,000 + 100,(+ 70,000) - 120,000 = 180,000 tablets.

EXAMPLE:

Table 8.4 shows the stock-card for paracetamol tablets 500 mg. Reading down the stock column we see that the main hospital stores ran out of stock of these tablets twice during the year. The first stockout occurred after the store issued the last 10,000 tablets to the hospital pharmacy on 20 January, and it lasted 9 days until 1 February, when 30,000 tablets were delivered from the central medical depot. It is unlikely that the pharmacy dispensed all the 10,000 tablets issued from the hospital store in only 9 days, and this is confirmed by the fact that the next issue from the store to the pharmacy was not made until 25 February. It is therefore safe to conclude that paracetamol tablets continued to be available in practice, so we may ignore the fact that the hospital store had a short stock-out.

The second stock-out lasted from 1 June until 31 July, that is 2 months. However, the 10,000 tablets issued on 1 June would have lasted for part of this time. Is it reasonable to use our rule of thumb and ignore the first month? To find out, we look at the quantities issued and the time periods between issues. The first issue was 10,000 tablets on 20 January; the second also of 10,000 tablets was 5 weeks later on 25 February; the third issue, again 10,000 tablets, was 7 weeks later on 20 April. Continuing in this way we see that 10,000 tablets last 5-7 weeks. It is therefore reasonable to say that the tablets were still actually available for at least a month after the last issue, and to count only the second month as a real stock-out.

Recorded consumption is 80,000 tablets.
Period in stock is 12 months minus 1 month effectively out of stock, which makes 11 months.
Calculation period is 12 months.

Applying the formula:

$$\text{Consumption adjusted for stock-outs} = 80{,}000 \text{ tab.} \times \frac{12 \text{ months}}{11 \text{ months}} = 87{,}273 \text{ tablets}$$

The answer is recorded in Table 8.6

Table 8.4
Illustrative stock cards

DRUG: PARACETAMOL TABLETS 500MG

CODE NUMBER: 02100501

DATE 1986		IN	OUT	STOCK
1 Jan	Opening stock			10 000
20 Jan	To hospital pharmacy		10 000	0
1 Feb	From central depot	30 000		30 000
25 Feb	To hospital phamacy		10 000	20 000
20 Apr	" "		10 000	10 000
1 Jun	" "		10 000	0
31 Jul	From central depot	50 000		50 000
1 Aug	To hospital pharmacy		10 000	40 000
7 Sep	" "		10 000	30 000
20 Oct	" "		10 000	20 000
10 Dec	" "		10 000	10 000
31 Dec	Closing stock			10 000

DRUG: CHLORPHENAMINE TABLETS 4MG

CODE NUMBER: 03000101

DATE 1986		IN	OUT	STOCK
1 Jan	Opening stock			2 000
15 Jan	To hospital pharmacy		1 000	1 000
15 Feb	" "		1 000	0
1 Mar	From central depot	5 000		5 000
10 Mar	To hospital pharmacy		1 000	4 000
7 Apr	" "		2 000	2 000
10 Jun	" "		1 000	1 000
7 Jul	" "		1 000	0
10 Oct	From central depot	5 000		5 000
11 Oct	To hospital pharmacy		2 000	3 000
30 Nov	" "		1 000	2 000
15 Dec	" "		1 000	1 000
31 Dec	Closing stock			1 000

EXERCISE 8C

Examine the stock-card for chlorphenamine tablets in Table 8.4 and answer the following questions:

1. **What is the recorded consumption of chlorphenamine?**
2. **Has the drug been out of stock?**
3. **If so, how long were the stock-out periods?**
4. **Which stock-outs require adjustments to be made?**
5. **What is the effective period during which the drug has been in stock?**
6. **What is the consumption adjusted for stock-outs?**

Check your answer at the foot of page 8.20 and in Table 8.6.

The adjustment for wastage and losses, and the adjustment for stock-outs have been explained separately for clarity. In practice, both adjustments may often be needed on the same stock card. This situation is illustrated in the following example.

Answer to exercise 8B:

1. The recorded consumption of sulfadimidine tablets 500mg is 72,000 tablets.
2. There are three items of avoidable wastage and losses:
   (a) 10 June: 7,000 tablets destroyed by damp
   (b) 20 Nov: 10,000 tablets destroyed because time-expired
   (c) 31 Dec: 5,000 tablets unaccounted for at end of year stock-taking
3. Adjusted consumption after allowing for avoidable wastage and losses is 72,000 - 22,000 = 50,000 tablets

EXAMPLE:

Table 8.5 shows the stock card for metrifonate tablets 100mg. Total recorded consumption is 17,000 tablets. However, we find that 2,000 tablets were destroyed by paraffin contamination in the stores on 5 March; when the last 1,000 tablets in stock were required for issue on 10 October, they could not be found. If we consider both these items as avoidable wastage and loss, then the real consumption is 17,000 – (2,000 + 1,000) = 14,000.

There have also been two stock-outs. The first was from 15 April to 8 June. Looking at the intervals between issues, it is reasonable to assume that the 1,000 tablets issued on 15 April would have lasted for 3-4 weeks. We therefore apply our rule of thumb and ignore the first month. This leaves an effective stock-out from 15 May - 8 June, that is roughly 3 weeks.

The second stock-out was from 10 October to 10 November. Applying our rule of thumb we should ignore this. However, like all rules of thumb it must be applied intelligently. The last issue of this drug was in fact on 30 August, and this would have been used up by 10 October, when it was discovered that 1,000 tablets supposed to be in stock were missing - presumably pilfered. The month's stock-out is therefore counted, for the drug was effectively out of stock. The period for which the drug was in stock is therefore 52 weeks - (3 weeks + 4 weeks) = 45 weeks.

Consumption adjusted for stock-outs = 14,000 x 52/45 = 16,178 tablets.

This answer is recorded in Table 8.6.

Table 8.5
Illustrative stock card

DRUG: METRIFONATE TABLETS 100MG

CODE NUMBER: 06800101

DATE	1986	IN	OUT	STOCK
1 Jan	Opening stock			1 000
5 Jan	From central depot	4 000		5 000
18 Jan	To hospital pharmacy		2 000	3 000
25 Feb	" "		1 000	2 000
5 Mar	From central depot	2 000		4 000
5 Mar	Contaminated (paraffin)		2 000	2 000
25 Mar	To hospital pharmacy		1 000	1 000
15 Apr	" "		1 000	0
8 Jun	From central depot	3 000		3 000
9 Jun	To hospital pharmacy		2 000	1 000
15 Jun	From central depot	4 000		5 000
20 Jul	To hospital pharmacy		2 000	3 000
30 Aug	" "		2 000	1 000
10 Oct	Unaccounted for		1 000	0
10 Nov	From central depot	4 000		4 000
11 Nov	To hospital pharmacy		2 000	2 000
15 Dec	" "		1 000	1 000
31 Dec	Closing stock			1 000

STEP 5: Calculate average drug use per 1,000 patient contacts.

We have now calculated the quantities of drugs consumed, but these are not very meaningful until we relate them to the workload of patients. If the facility we are dealing with has only out-patient activities, we simply divide the adjusted consumption of each drug by the total number of out-patient consultations.

EXAMPLE:

Returning to the illustrative stock-card in Tables 8.3 and 8.4, we know that the annual consumption of lidocaine 1% 50 ml vials is 120 per year. Suppose this "standard" facility had 60,000 out-patient consultations during the year. Then:

$$\text{Average consumption} = \frac{120 \text{ vials}}{60 \text{ thousand contacts}} = 2 \text{ vials per } 1{,}000 \text{ patient contacts}$$

This calculation is appropriate for a facility having only out-patients. However, the "standard" facility we are using for illustration is a hospital, which also treats in-patients. How are these to be taken into account? Field tests of this manual have shown that the consumption expressed per 1,000 out-patient consultations provides a reliable indication of the total quantity of drugs required, including a proportion for in-patients, **but only if the ratio of in-patient admissions to out-patient consultations is relatively uniform in all facilities of the type concerned.**

EXAMPLE:

Suppose that our "standard" hospital had 60,000 out-patient consultations, and 6,000 in-patient admissions during the year, this gives a ratio of 100 admissions per 1,000 out-patient consultations. Our calculation of 2 vials of lidocaine per 1,000 out-patient consultations would therefore include the consumption by 100 in-patients.

If, in another hospital, we found 30,000 out-patient consultations and 3,000 in-patient admissions, the ratio is still 100 admissions per 1,000 out-patient consultations, so 2 vials of lidocaine per 1,000 out-patient consultations will again be sufficient for the in-patients at this hospital.

Now, suppose that in a third hospital we find 30,000 out-patient consultations and 6,000 in-patient admissions. This gives a ratio of 200 admissions per 1,000 consultations. Our estimate of 2 vials of lidocaine per 1,000 out-patients allow for only 100 in-patients, and may therefore be insufficient.

Table 8.6
Calculation sheet for recording drug quantities (consumption method)

	drug generic name	dosage form and strength	Drug use per year	Period the drug was out of stock during the year	Adjusted consumption per year	Number of outpatients per year	Average drug consumption per 1000 outpat.
A	acetylsalicylic acid	tab 300 mg	180,000				
	aluminium hydroxide	tab 500 mg					
	aluminium acetate	drp 13% ml					
	antivenom sera	inj IV 100 ml					
	ampicillin	cap 250 mg					
B	benzath benzylpenic	inj 2.4 MU vial					
	benzoic & sal. acid	oint 6% & 3% mg					
	benzyl benzoate	sol 25% ml					
C	calamine lotion	lot ml					
	chloramphenicol	cap 250 mg					
	chloramphenicol	inj 1 g amp					
	chlorhexidine	sol conc 5% ml					
	chloroquine	tab 150 mg base					
	chlorphenamine	tab 4 mg	11,000	65 days	13383	60000	223
	chlorpromazine	tab 100 mg					
D	dapsone	tab 50 mg					
	dextran 70	inj sol 6% 500ml					
	diazepam	tab 5 mg					
	diazepam	inj 10mg/2ml vial					
	diethylcarbamazine	tab 50 mg					
E	epinephrine	inj 1 mg/ml amp					
	ergometrine	inj 0.2 mg/ml amp					

continued

Table 8.6 (continued)

	drug generic name	dosage form and strength	Drug use per year	Period the drug was out of stock during the year	Adjusted consumption per year	Number of outpatients per year	Average drug consumption per 1000 outpat.
F	ferrous sulfate	tab 60 mg					
	fer.sulf & fol.ac.	tab 60 mg & 0.25 mg					
	fluoresceine	drps eye 1% 1 ml					
	folic acid	tab 1 mg					
G	gentian violet	crystal mg					
	glibenclamide	tab 4 mg					
	glyceryl trinitrate	tab 25 mg					
H	hydrochlorothiazide	tab 25 mg					
I	imipramine	tab 25 mg					
	insulin zc sus comp	inj 40 IU/ml, 10 ml					
	ipecacuanha	syr 0.14% ml					
L	lidocaine	inj sol 1% 50 ml	120	0	120	60000	2
	lindane	lot 1% ml					
M	mebendazole	tab 100 mg					
	metrifonate	tab 100 mg	14,000	7 weeks	16178	60000	270
	metronidazole	tab 200 mg					
N	neomyc bacitracin	oin 5 mg&500 IU, 20g					
	niclosamide	tab 500 mg					
	nystatin	pes 100,000 IU					
O	oral rehydr salts	pkt 1 litre					
	oxamniquine	cap 250 mg					
P	paracetamol	tab 500 mg	80,000	1 month	87273	60000	1455
	pethidine	inj 100 mg/2ml amp					
	phenobarbital	tab 50 mg					
	phenytoin	tab 100 mg					

continued

Table 8.6 (continued)

	drug generic name	dosage form and strength	Drug use per year	Period the drug was out of stock during the year	Adjusted consumption per year	Number of outpatients per year	Average drug consumption per 1000 outpat.
	phenoxymeth penicil	tab 250 mg					
	praziquantel	tab 600 mg					
	probenecid	tab 500 mg					
	proc benzylpenicil	inj 3 MU vial	4,200		4200	60000	70
	promethazine	tab 25 mg					
Q	quinine	tab 300 mg					
	quinine	inj 300 mg/ml, 2ml					
R	Ringers solution	sol 500 ml					
S	salbutamol	tab 4 mg					
	senna	tab 7.5 mg					
	spectinomycin	inj 2 g vial					
	streptomycin	inj 1 g vial					
	sulfadimadine	tab 500 mg	50,000		50000	60000	833
	sulfameth/trimethopr.	tab 400 mg & 80 mg					
	suramin sodium	inj 1 g vial					
T	tetracycline	cap 250 mg					
	tetracycline	oin eye 1% tube 5 g					
	thiacetazone/INH	tab 150 mg & 300 mg					
V	vitamin A (retinol)	cap 200 000 IU					
W	water for injection	10 ml amp					

If the ratio of in-patient admissions to out-patient consultations varies considerably between the hospitals whose drug needs are being estimated, then both elements need to be included in the calculation, otherwise the estimates will not be reliable. The ideal solution in such cases is to estimate in-patient and out-patient drug consumption separately. Hospitals may not keep separate records for in-patient and out-patient drug consumption, so the data will not be available.

The next best solution is to combine out-patient consultations and in-patient admissions to a single denominator. The simplest way to do this would be to add together admissions and consultations, but such an addition is valid only if the drug consumption per out-patient consultation is roughly the same as for an in-patient stay. This might occur in lower level facilities such as health centres with a few beds. However, it is unlikely in larger hospitals providing relatively sophisticated in-patient services to more serious cases. For these we must estimate the ratio of the average use of drugs consumed per in-patient admission to the average use of drugs consumed per out-patient consultation. This ratio may be estimated subjectively on the basis of the clinical opinion of the medical staff at the facilities concerned, but it is usually safer also to review a sample of in-patient and out-patient records to obtain a more objective basis of estimation.

EXAMPLE:

Our "standard" hospital has 60,000 out-patient consultations and 6,000 in-patient admissions. If the average consumption is about the same for each one then we simply add the two to obtain the denominator of 66,000 patient contacts. However, if it is estimated that the average quantity of drugs consumed per in-patient case is three times more than for an out-patient consultation, then we multiply the 6,000 in-patients by three before we add them to the out-patient consultations, so the final denominator is 60,000 + 18,000 = 78,000 patient contacts.

STEP 6: Consolidate the answers from all the "standard" facilities in the sample.

The reliability and predictive value of the consumption method increases when drug consumption at more than one health facility is taken as the basis for the estimations. In step 5 we have calculated average drug use per thousand patient contacts for one such health facility. After the consumption of drugs in one facility has been calculated, it is advisable to collect data from a few similar facilities and calculate the drug use per thousand patient contacts for all the "standard" facilities together.

STEP 7: Scale up the answer from the sample to cover all facilities.

We now have estimated drug requirements per 1,000 patient contacts (see Column 7 of Table 8.6). In order to convert this into an estimate for all the facilities, each drug quantity must be multiplied by the expected number of patient contacts in thousands at the facilities covered by the quantification.

EXAMPLE:

> ***Suppose it is estimated that 1,200 acetylsalicylic acid tablets 300mg are required per 1,000 patient contacts, and it is estimated that the facilities to be covered by the quantification will have 594,000 patient contacts. Then the total quantity required will be 1,200 x 594 = 712,800 tablets. As acetylsalicylic acid tablets are supplied in tins of thousand tablets (see Table 4.8) 713 tins will be needed (see also Task 12, step 4, on page 7.16).***

After task 12, the calculation continues with tasks 13-17 (page 7.15). These are identical for both quantification methods, and they have been explained in Modules 3 and 7.

Answer to exercise 8C:

1. The recorded consumption of chlorphenamine is 11,000 tablets.
2. Yes, there have been two stock-outs.
3. First from 15 February to 1 March (14 days)
   Second from 7 July to 10 October = 95 days (24 days of July + 31 for August + 30 for September + 9 days in October).
4. The first stock-out can be ignored (the stock card shows that 1,000 chlorphenamine tablets normally last at least a month). Ignoring the first month, according to our rule of thumb, the second stock-out lasted 65 days, and an adjustment is required.
5. Chlorphenamine has been in stock for 365 - 65 = 300 days.
6. Adjusted consumption is:

$$11{,}000 \text{ tablets} \times \frac{365 \text{ days}}{300 \text{ days}} = 13{,}383 \text{ tablets}$$

If you measured the stock-out more approximately in months, 7 July to 10 October is roughly three months. Since we can ignore the first month, the effective stock-out is 2 months. Then adjusted consumption =

$$11{,}000 \text{ tablets} \times \frac{12 \text{ months}}{10 \text{ months}} = 13{,}200 \text{ tablets}$$

ANNEXES

Annex 1
Model record form for the community health worker

Name: Location:

1 ICD Code	2 Health problem	3 :Children under 5 :	4 Total	5 :Children five and over, & adults :	6 Total	7 : TOTAL
009.2	Acute diarrhoea: Severity 1	:00000 00000 00000:		:00000 00000 00000 00000 00000 00000:		:
	Severity 2:	:00000 00000 00000:		:00000 00000 00000 00000 00000 00000:		:
	Severity 3:	:00000 00000 00000:		:00000 00000 00000 00000 00000 00000:		:
084	Malaria - Severity 1	:00000 00000 00000:		:00000 00000 00000 00000 00000 00000:		:
		:00000 00000 00000:		:00000 00000 00000 00000 00000 00000:		:
127.0	Ascariasis (roundworm)	:00000 00000 00000:		:00000 00000 00000 00000 00000 00000:		:
		:00000 00000 00000:		:00000 00000 00000 00000 00000 00000:		:
132	Pediculosis (lice)	:00000 00000 00000:		:00000 00000 00000 00000 00000 00000:		:
133.0	Scabies	:00000 00000 00000:		:00000 00000 00000 00000 00000 00000:		:
280	Iron deficiency anaemia	:00000 00000 00000:		:00000 00000 00000 00000 00000 00000:		:
372.0	Conjunctivitis	:00000 00000 00000:		:00000 00000 00000 00000 00000 00000:		:
460	Common cold	:00000 00000 00000:		:00000 00000 00000 00000 00000 00000:		:
521.0	Caries, toothache	:00000 00000 00000:		:00000 00000 00000 00000 00000 00000:		:
535-6	Gastritis, heartburn, indigestion	:00000 00000 00000:		:00000 00000 00000 00000 00000 00000:		:
564.0	Constipation	:00000 00000 00000:		:00000 00000 00000 00000 00000 00000:		:
595	Cystitis: Severity 1	:00000 00000 00000:		:00000 00000 00000 00000 00000 00000:		:
	Severity 2	:00000 00000 00000:		:00000 00000 00000 00000 00000 00000:		:
680-2	Boil, abscess	:00000 00000 00000:		:00000 00000 00000 00000 00000 00000:		:
684	Impetigo, bacterial skin infection	:00000 00000 00000:		:00000 00000 00000 00000 00000 00000:		:
714-6	Chronic arthritis and arthrosis	:00000 00000 00000:		:00000 00000 00000 00000 00000 00000:		:
724	Back-pain, lumbago	:00000 00000 00000:		:00000 00000 00000 00000 00000 00000:		:
780.6	Fever NEC	:00000 00000 00000:		:00000 00000 00000 00000 00000 00000:		:
780.7	Malaise, fatigue NEC	:00000 00000 00000:		:00000 00000 00000 00000 00000 00000:		:
784.0	Headache NEC	:00000 00000 00000:		:00000 00000 00000 00000 00000 00000:		:
786.2	Cough NEC	:00000 00000 00000:		:00000 00000 00000 00000 00000 00000:		:
789.0	Abdominal pain NEC	:00000 00000 00000:		:00000 00000 00000 00000 00000 00000:		:
840-8	Sprains and strains	:00000 00000 00000:		:00000 00000 00000 00000 00000 00000:		:
910-19	Superficial injury, bruise, cut	:00000 00000 00000:		:00000 00000 00000 00000 00000 00000:		:
940-9	Burns	:00000 00000 00000:		:00000 00000 00000 00000 00000 00000:		:
		TOTAL A:		TOTAL A :		:
REPEAT VISITS FOR SAME HEALTH PROBLEM						
	Injections	:00000 00000 00000:		:00000 00000 00000 00000 00000 00000:		:
	Dressings	:00000 00000 00000:		:00000 00000 00000 00000 00000 00000:		:
	Oral medication	:00000 00000 00000:		:00000 00000 00000 00000 00000 00000:		:
	Follow-up visit	:00000 00000 00000:		:00000 00000 00000 00000 00000 00000:		:
		TOTAL B:		TOTAL B :		:
		TOTAL A+B:		TOTAL A+B :		:
OTHER HEALTH SERVICE CONTACTS						
V03-06	Vaccinations	:00000 00000 00000:		:00000 00000 00000 00000 00000 00000:		:
		:00000 00000 00000:		:00000 00000 00000 00000 00000 00000:		:
V20	Under-five preventative care	:00000 00000 00000:				:
		:00000 00000 00000:				:
V22-3	Antenatal care			:00000 00000 00000 00000 00000 00000:		:
				:00000 00000 00000 00000 00000 00000:		:
V25	Family planning, contraception			:00000 00000 00000 00000 00000 00000:		:
				:00000 00000 00000 00000 00000 00000:		:
V70	Medical examination, no illness	:00000 00000 00000:		:00000 00000 00000 00000 00000 00000:		:
		TOTAL C:		TOTAL C :		:
		TOTAL A+B+C:		TOTAL A+B+C :		:

Annex 2
Calculation sheet for drug quantities by health problem

1 ICD Code	2 Health problem	3 Standard treatment Drug generic name, dosage form and strength	4 Quantity per standard treatment	5 Number of treatment episodes	6 TOTAL QUANTITY

Annex 3
Calculation sheet for total quantities of each drug, number of order packs and cost

1 Drug code number	2 Drug generic name, dosage form and strength	3 ICD code of health problem for which indicated & severity & age group	4 Total quantity for all standard treatments (in counting units)	5 Total quantity including allowance for wastage & loss	6 Order pack size = (number of units / pack)	7 Number of packs required (rounded to the nearest whole number)	8 Price per pack ($)	9 Total cost	10 Percent of total cost

Annex 4
Calculation sheet for total drug quantities and cost after reconciliation to budget, and quantities per 1000 treatment episodes

1 Drug generic name, dosage form and strength	2 Number of packs required (rounded to the nearest whole number)	3 Price per pack $	4 Total cost $	5 Percent of total cost:	6 Final number of packs required adjusted to budget:	7 Pack size: (in counting units)	8 TOTAL COST ($)	9 Final: quantity (in counting units)	10 Number of counting units per 1000 treatment episodes

Annex 5
Calculation sheet for recording drug quantities (consumption method)

Drug generic name	Dosage form and strength	Drug use per year	Period the drug was out of stock during the year	Adjusted consumption per year	Number of outpatients per year	Average drug consumption per 1000 outpat.
aluminium hydroxide	tab 500 mg					
aluminium acetate	drp 13% ml					
antivenom sera	inj IV 100 ml					
ampicillin	cap 250 mg					
benzath benzylpenic	inj 2.4 MU vial					
benzoic & sal. acid	oint 6% & 3% mg					
benzyl benzoate	sol 25% ml					
calamine lotion	lot ml					
chloramphenicol	cap 250 mg					
chloramphenicol	inj 1 g amp					
chlorhexidine	sol conc 5% ml					
chloroquine	tab 150 mg base					
chlorphenamine	tab 4 mg					
chlorpromazine	tab 100 mg					
dapsone	tab 50 mg					
dextran 70	inj sol 6% 500ml					
diazepam	tab 5 mg					
diazepam	inj 10mg/2ml vial					
diethylcarbamazine	tab 50 mg					
epinephrine	inj 1 mg/ml amp					
ergometrine	inj 0.2 mg/ml amp					

Annex 5 (continued)

Drug generic name	Dosage form and strength	Drug use per year	Period the drug was out of stock during the year	Adjusted consumption per year	Number of outpatients per year	Average drug consumption per 1000 outpat.
ferrous sulfate	tab 60 mg					
fer.sulf & fol.ac.	tab 60 mg & 0.25 mg					
fluoresceine	drps eye 1% 1 ml					
folic acid	tab 1 mg					
gentian violet	crystal mg					
glibenclamide	tab 4 mg					
glyceryl trinitrate	tab 25 mg					
hydrochlorothiazide	tab 25 mg					
imipramine	tab 25 mg					
insulin zc sus comp	inj 40 IU/ml, 10 ml					
ipecacuanha	syr 0.14% ml:					
lidocaine	inj sol 1% 50 ml					
lindane	lot 1% ml					
mebendazole	tab 100 mg					
metrifonate	tab 100 mg					
metronidazole	tab 200 mg					
neomyc bacitracin	oin 5 mg&500 IU, 20g					
niclosamide	tab 500 mg					
nystatin	pes 100,000 IU					
oral rehydr salts	pkt 1 litre					
oxamniquine	cap 250 mg					
paracetamol	tab 500 mg					
pethidine	inj 100 mg/2ml amp					
phenobarbital	tab 50 mg					
phenytoin	tab 100 mg					

Annex 5 (continued)

Drug generic name	Dosage form and strength	Drug use per year	Period the drug was out of stock during the year	Adjusted consumption per year	Number of outpatients per year	Average drug consumption per 1000 outpat.
phenoxymeth penicil	tab 250 mg					
praziquantel	tab 600 mg					
probenecid	tab 500 mg					
proc benzylpenicil	inj 3 MU vial					
promethazine	tab 25 mg					
quinine	tab 300 mg					
quinine	inj 300 mg/ml, 2ml					
Ringers solution	sol 500 ml					
salbutamol	tab 4 mg					
senna	tab 7.5 mg					
spectinomycin	inj 2 g vial					
streptomycin	inj 1 g vial					
sulfadimadine	tab 500 mg					
sulfameth/trimethopr.	tab 400 mg & 80 mg					
suramin sodium	inj 1 g vial					
tetracycline	cap 250 mg					
tetracycline	oin eye 1% tube 5 g					
thiacetazone/INH	tab 150 mg & 300 mg					
vitamin A (retinol)	cap 200 000 IU					
water for injection	10 ml amp					